My name is John E. Med..., ... 37 years old, living in Cincinnati, Ohio. In 2004, I graduated from The University of Dayton, where I earned a degree in psychology.

I was first diagnosed with bipolar one disorder with psychotic features in July of 2006. This is just when I was diagnosed. I believe that I showed symptoms long before 2006, perhaps most of my life.

Since then, Panic Disorder, Obsessive Compulsive Disorder, Post Traumatic Stress Disorder, and Generalized Anxiety Disorder have been added to my complete diagnosis. I also have trouble with confined spaces (claustrophobia) and wide open spaces (agoraphobia).

When I started to feel better and coherent, I knew that I wanted to help others in a similar situation. I started a social media page called Mental Health Awareness and Online Support, and there are almost 700 members now. I have written two books already. One is my life story titled, "Millions Like Me: My Struggle with Mental Illness" and the other is a book of poetry titled, "Poems from a Bipolar Mind". I hope that this book will tie everything together.

The most important thing I want to convey to you is that you are not alone. Mental illness is fairly common, but unfortunately, not a lot of people talk about it because of the stigma that is attached to it. I talk about it a lot, and so do many others. It's okay to not be okay sometimes. It takes incredible courage to face mental illness every day. Feel free to look me up on social media or join my page if you have no other support. I consider myself a survivor and a success story at this point.

January 2, 2019

I had a realization today. An epiphany, if you will. I don't know everything, and I make mistakes. Shocking, right? I've probably done a lot of things the wrong way, and I've made some bad choices. I've made a lot of good choices too, and I've done a lot of good with what I have. That's life and part of being human I guess. I feel like most of the time I've tried my best, and at the end of the day, that's all I can expect of myself.

January 4, 2019

Mental health professionals say all the time, "You are not your illness", but where do I draw the line of taking responsibility for my actions? What is my personality and what is my illness? Is it both? Was I just an active child that played sports and excelled at school or was that the beginning of mania? When I went on road trips to concerts and experimented with drugs, was I just having fun and being rebellious or was that my illness? Was I having fun or self medicating? When I was working 60+ hours a week and going to college full-time, was I manic or just showing a good work ethic? I fully believe in taking responsibility for my actions, but the line is blurry. There are times in my life where I can definitely say, "Okay, my mind wasn't right. I was going through psychosis and insanity", but the rest is kind of up for debate. I guess it doesn't matter now because the only reason I want to know what I am responsible for is so that I can feel guilty about it, which doesn't do anyone any good.

January 6, 2019

It was a challenge to work full time and get a college degree, but even that was only for 4 years. I'm going on 13 years dealing with mental illness, and it's frustrating and exhausting at times. My mood has been all over the place for weeks, but mostly sad and exhausted. I think I just need some direction or a new project to put my energy into. I always feel like the end game is for me to get a job/career and move out on my own, but what if it's not? Am I going to be on disability and live with family the rest of my life? I run out of patience a lot with myself, and I get bored easily. It wouldn't be so bad if I could concentrate enough to read a book or write or something. I can't just sit around and be exhausted and think about my troubles. This isn't normal. This isn't how healthy brains work. I know a lot of people will try to explain it away with the usual stuff, but all this is absolutely my mental illness. It's hard to even explain to people who don't have it. I think my doctor and case manager understand pretty well for not having a mental illness, but I don't know how much other people really understand how hard it is.

January 8, 2019

7 Goals for the near future (into 2019):

1) Continue to lose weight by making healthy food choices and having food portion discipline.
2) Realize that I cannot help or please everyone.
3) Continue to test my anxiety, but also realize that sometimes I just want the peace of my home.
4) Love myself, which in part means forgiving myself for the mistakes I have made and the time I have wasted on people who used me.
5) Strive for 100% effort.
6) Continue helping others, but also setting limits where I may

need to take a break and rest. The weight of the world is not mine to bear, and other people's problems are not mine either. I need to use discretion when helping others and set healthy boundaries.

7) Practice gratitude and mindfulness on the days when I am depressed, and when negativity crosses my path.

January 11, 2019

I still remember. Eighth floor. East wing at University Hospital in Cincinnati. Also known as "Beast". It would be my home for almost two weeks in 2006. Locked down until I was no longer a threat to myself or anyone else. Before I was escorted to this wing of the hospital, I was given an injection that calmed me down, and I slept for several hours. I have a few triggers that take me back to that time. A scene from a medical TV show or movie. Maybe a prescription drug commercial. When I have to see the doctor like I have to tomorrow. I have flashbulb memories of a large syringe. It's like a picture card in my mind that flashes when I am triggered. It comes and goes, but the memories have never completely disappeared. I still remember what the inside of the community shower looked like. I remember reading the Bible to my friends that came to visit, and thinking that I could predict the end of the world. I remember my visitors sneaking in non-hospital food for me. I remember ripping the bulletin board off the wall because I thought there was a secret tunnel behind it.

January 13, 2019

Today was the last day that I had to see my current, and now former, doctor. I feel like I have a pretty good plan in place, and no medication changes or anything. I have made a lot of progress under his treatment. I remember when I could barely ride in a car, not even being the driver because of my anxiety. I did really well today. Not much anxiety at all. In the past, sometimes I couldn't sit still in the waiting room or the doctor's office because my chest hurt so badly from anxiety or I would get dizzy spells. Losing about 60-70 pounds has definitely helped too. I only weigh myself about 5 times a year because I don't want to obsess about a number. The reason I weigh myself is simply to track progress. Just a measuring stick type thing. I will probably only have to see the doctor every 2-4 months now, instead of every month, assuming there are no medication or condition changes. I'm really happy about that. I felt like my freedom was being taken away when I had to see the doctor every month. I don't have to report back until February 27th!

January 14, 2019

Most days, all I ask of myself is to give my best effort. I try not to focus on results, because sometimes the effort is there, but the results are not. If I can get through a day with minimal symptoms, and accomplish a few simple tasks, that's a good day for me. Arguably, a great day. Any advocacy work that I accomplish is a bonus too. I try to help others whenever I can.

January 16, 2019

I remember in high school I had an assignment where I was supposed to write about what kind of career I wanted. The idea was to start to think about possible majors in college and a career. I was honest and wrote that I didn't care what I did for a living as long as I was happy. There's rumors that John Lennon wrote something similar. I just didn't see the point of having money and all the finer things in life if I wasn't happy. I still don't care too much for money. It's simply a means to an end. The world runs on money, so I try to make it, but in the end, money doesn't buy my health and happiness.

January 17, 2019

I avoid watching the news, but it's hard because I live with my parents who are of the older persuasion. It seems like every story, except the weather, is negative and disturbing. I live in Ohio, so sometimes even the weather is depressing. I know that bad things happen in the world, but I just chose to avoid hearing about it through the news. The problem I have is that, as an empathetic person, I feel pain and sadness. Literally feel it physically. If I hear too much sad or disturbing news in a short time, it affects my mood too. Avoiding the news for me is almost a means of survival.

January 18, 2019

Mental illness is one of those things that most people don't care about until it happens to them or it hits close to home. I guess a lot of things are like that. I try my best to help people who are receptive, understand, but I'm starting to think that no one truly understands until it happens to him/her. God bless the people who love and support me even though they might not completely understand. Even after 13 years, members of my own family don't try to understand, or they are just incapable. People would rather ignore it and hope it gets better or disappears. Mental illness isn't going anywhere, and if I had to guess, the numbers of people affected is just going to grow.

January 20, 2019

I started playing Texas Hold 'Em Poker when I was 18 years old. I thought some day I might be a professional player. I still haven't completely given up on that dream. I joined a card club many years ago, but I haven't been able to play regularly in recent years because of my anxiety and depression. The club meets every other Friday, so there are a lot of events in a year. I would sit home on those Fridays and wish I could play and enjoy myself like I used to. Last night, I took the leap and drove 15-20 minutes to the host's house. I stayed and played cards all night, with very little problems. This was a huge accomplishment for me, and it is keeping me hopeful that I can get better. With anxiety and depression, sometimes you reach a breaking point. You would rather fail than stay in the same condition of misery. That's what happened. I had enough. Now I feel like I accomplished something, and I had fun along the way.

January 21, 2019

It's January here in Ohio. We just had a snow storm that dumped about 10 inches of snow on us over a weekend. When snow happens, our driveway and walkway needs to be cleared with a shovel. I was able to help my dad clear the way this year, which I was not able to do last year. I can't remember if I was unsteady because of anxiety or my body weight, but I am almost 70 pounds lighter, and I am managing my anxiety better. I was a little worried that I wouldn't be able to help again because of body soreness, but I just drank a cup of coffee and went for it. Sometimes I feel so helpless because I can't help out with daily chores, but I am making progress in that area. I feel better about myself the more active and productive I am, and it gives me hope that I will just keep being able to do more and more.

January 22, 2019

This is something strange about me that I think about a lot. I really can't figure it out. I used to drink alcohol and smoke weed every day. I think it was how I used to cope with my illness. But then, after I was diagnosed at age 24, I continued to self-medicate with booze and weed. Now, I am sober 99.9% of the time, and I rarely feel the need to have a drink or smoke anymore. It's like my cravings for those substances just disappeared. If I had a drinking or smoking problem, I would think it would have been harder for me to stop. Maybe it's a testament to the effectiveness of my medication. I think in the end, being sober is a blessing. I can't afford it anyway, and I respect my parents to the point that I don't want to be all messed up while they are letting me live with them. Maybe that's why I don't do it anymore. I've always been very confused about this.

January 23, 2019

With mental illness comes side effects of medications and symptoms of the actual illness. The medical field tries to quantify and name all of these feelings, but sometimes I just feel weird and awful. I'm sure if I thought hard about it, I could give these feelings a name. Maybe it's when multiple symptoms and side effects hit me all at once. I just feel a little off sometimes, but these moments are getting less and less frequent over the years. I remember one night I was laying in bed, and I just felt terrible. I think it was mainly anxiety and panic, but it was just an awful weird feeling. I text messaged all my loved ones and told them I loved them and that I might not make it through the night. That's how convinced I was that I might actually die. This was several years ago, and I haven't really felt awful to that degree in quite a while. One thing I took away from that night was to (try) and not take a day for granted, and I tell my loved ones that I love them on a regular basis. I just don't want there to be any doubt if anything should happen to me. I know this is completely overdoing it, but anxiety and panic and all the other symptoms make it seem reasonable and logical. I don't think "overloving" people is such a bad thing anyway.

January 24, 2019

I get up for the day anywhere between 2-4AM. Sometimes I sleep. Sometimes I don't at all. I have some coffee and attend to messages and emails and such. Sometimes I play computer games. I am the creator and administrator of a free social media page called Mental Health Awareness and Online Support also. I constantly work on that every day. I don't know if I've ever taken a day off in the last 7 years. I post mainly inspirational material, but sometimes personal thoughts or interesting articles I find about coping with mental illness. I take some medication at 4AM and eat a small breakfast, and then it's back to bed for me until about 10AM.

January 25, 2019

Sometimes when I get anxious or when I'm having a panic attack, it helps me to look into my eyes in the mirror. I get this fierce feeling like I am going to keep fighting. In reality, I think it is a form of grounding, which is a technique used to calm a person down by being aware of things that can be experienced with the five senses. It's more romantic to think of this fighting spirit as an X factor or "wow" factor. The kind of intangible spirit that sports broadcasters talk about in a winning athlete. That's how I like to think about it anyway.

Most days, when I wake up in the morning, I am very lethargic. I can't wait to get to the coffee pot. Same goes for any time I take a nap. To my credit, I always get up. There was one day a few years ago where I just couldn't do it that day, and I stayed in bed all day. Some nights, I don't sleep at all, usually when I have a lot on my mind or have an obligation the next day. There are very few days when I wake up well rested and refreshed, but today is one of those days. It will probably last until I take my first dose of medicine, so I wanted to do some writing before that happens.

Today it was like I was shot out of a cannon when I woke up. These days are rare. We had a snow storm here in Ohio last night, and I am anxious to shovel the snow and clear the walkway and driveway. I think that's why I have this unexplainable energy. Such is the life of a bipolar person with anxiety.

It seems to me that there are essentially two choices when deciding on a career path. You can either go for money or serve others because there aren't many professions that both pay a lot and allow someone to help others. I think it's a shame, and I know that's probably simplifying things, but it's an explanation I have thought about as to why teachers for example are paid so little and doctors, lawyers, and politicians are paid exorbitant amounts of money. Then you have the rare breed of people who do well for themselves financially and give back to their communities or charities. I think that's how I want to be. I really just want enough money to live comfortably and help my family, and hopefully there would be some left over to do some good in the world. I'm not the type of person who really enjoys luxury. I have never really understood why people spend so much money on material things. I don't know what good a nice car would be to me when I can barely drive because of my anxiety. I would much rather be mentally stable and healthy than just about anything else.

I'm always a little proud of myself when I effectively manage my anxiety without having to take my medication "early". Early in quotes because my doctor says to take my anxiety medication (Klonopin) as needed, but my OCD nature has created a strict schedule. I just feel off for the day if I deviate from that schedule.

The amazing thing to me about anxiety are the physical symptoms. I think a lot of people think that anxiety and panic are just feelings or emotions. I wish that's all there was to it. Physical symptoms that I experience are: dizziness, foggy thoughts, tingling in my limbs, heart palpitations, nausea, sweating, chest pains, and muscle soreness/tension. As you could imagine, anxiety and panic are a lot harder to deal with when you take into account these physical symptoms. If anxiety and panic were just feelings, I think I wouldn't have nearly as much trouble overcoming triggers and uncomfortable situations. Sometimes the physical pain is overwhelming, and I have to lay down to make the soreness go away, and then that usually leads to a nap. When I take a brief nap, my symptoms "reset" as I like to say. Everything goes away for a short time, and I start a new battle when I wake up.

I have found several social media posts and other random thoughts that I have posted, so the linear dates are out of whack for a few pages.

Mania is defined as "mental illness marked by periods of great excitement, euphoria, delusions, and over activity." and "an excessive enthusiasm or desire; an obsession". It is the defining feature of bipolar disorder. Some bipolar sufferers have more mania than depression (bipolar one) or some have more depression than mania (bipolar two), but mania is always present. It can last hours, days, months, or years. I am writing this to exhaust the mania I am feeling right now. Mania can cause extreme productivity, but it can also be destructive in the form of poor choices. I am trying to use my energy right now in a productive way. I think of mania as a green light, and I have anxiety, which I think of as a stop sign. I experience both at the same time, so maybe you can imagine the confusion it causes in my mind and body. Sometimes, I want to drive across the country, for example, but my anxiety says no. Very frustrating. I end up just spinning my proverbial tires.

Earlier today, I made a careless mistake. I had coffee AFTER taking my medication when I know that I can only have coffee BEFORE I take my medication. I basically make myself get "up" with caffeine, and my medication brings me down to make me even overall. It's been this way for years. A substance as seemingly harmless as caffeine really affects me. I know better. Let's be honest here. My life would probably be more stable if I gave up caffeine all together, but I'm not willing to be sedated and tired all the time. The result was several panic attacks and about 4 hours of general anxiety. I refuse to take extra medication, so I just battled until it was over. I just kept telling myself over and over that my symptoms would go away. Eventually they did, but 4 hours is a long time to have anxiety, and my ego and confidence is bruised. I beat myself up for hours, and I honestly hated myself. I thought about all the mistakes and poor choices I've made in my past. I had chest pains and I was sweating. My whole body was sore. In order to remain somewhat stable, my illness requires my full attention and care. I failed today.

If you don't think anyone cares about you, I care. You matter. The world would be completely different without you. Yes, we are insignificant individually in a way, but that doesn't mean you can't make an impact. Everyone is worth saving who wants to be. You have to want it. Effort is an ability that everyone has. It doesn't matter where you come from or what has happened to you. Some days, I don't give my best effort, but I try. If you fail or stumble, don't give up. You just have to keep trying. Over and over. There's dignity in that I think. At the end of the day, people will respect you and your story will inspire others to keep trying in the face of adversity. I'm so blessed that I have a safe place to live and much support from friends, relatives, and even strangers. I try to pay that back by being there for others. There are a lot of people who dedicate their lives to helping others. They are just waiting to help you if you need it.

Letter to the doctor in 2013:

Mentally, I am pretty stable most days. I have some hypomanic episodes mixed with some depressive episodes. Lately, I have had a few depressive episodes where I just laid in bed and felt like I couldn't move, with some crying mixed in. I had a few days of racing thoughts in the last couple months where my brain wouldn't shut up, and it completely exhausts me. I get frustrated because I get anxious when I think about leaving the house sometimes, and it seems impossible for me to travel any amount of distance from home. Most times, I don't go places with any substantial number of people either. I also get frustrated because sometimes I feel stuck in a rut of not really happy, but not really sad either. I think you told me one time that people with bipolar disorder hate moderation and stability, so I guess that fits, and bipolar disorder is a disorder of extremes after all (the "dog bone" model we have talked about). What I mean by a dog bone is that there are knots on the end of a dog bone, with an even rod in the middle. My doctor aims to keep me on the middle rod, and not on one of the knobs/extremes. I haven't had any really serious panic attacks for quite some time, but I tend to be fidgety on occasion. Ironically, the most anxiety I get is when I have to see you, or have some other appointment, so I tend to avoid them. I realize that this is not your fault, and I have told you I like you as my doctor.

Physically, I am still trying to diet, and I have kept off 65 pounds since 2009, but I have been lighter. I am working on losing weight still. Minor aches and pains tend to ramp up my anxiety as well. I do a lot of activities on the computer, so my neck, wrists, shoulders, and arms get stiff sometimes. Sometimes, if I sit a certain way, my arms and/or legs will get pins and needles. It always seems to be my left side though. I think it is just the way I sit on the couch with my leg underneath me. My sleeping schedule is frustrating, and it goes something like this: 1am-4am, 9am-noon, 2pm-4:30pm. I don't know if I am satisfied with this, and I don't know if it's "normal" for someone like me, considering the medications I am on. I feel like if I wake up too far away from my medication times, I will get anxious. My medication times are 5am, noon, 5pm, and 10pm with little variation. On the rare occasion I go out, I can hold off on the night meds until later. Or by the off chance I sleep later, I can take my morning meds later, but it is very rare. I drink coffee and smoke cigarettes, and I hate to admit it, but I am addicted to the small "upper" feelings I get from the combination. I rarely drink alcohol, but it seems to take away all the symptoms for the time being. The after effects are what usually keep me from drinking. For example, in the morning, I may be more anxious, or just feel disconnected.

Why is mental illness so exhausting?

So I read a few articles about this because I never really educated myself on this topic. I just always feel exhausted, and I wondered if it was a lack of effort or because of my weight or what. Here's what I found:

1) The psychiatric medications often cause fatigue
2) Sleep disturbances-- too much or too little
3) Recovery takes a huge amount of mental and physical energy
4) Learning about and practicing self care

"I write about self-care, touch on it at the least, in pretty much every blog. And it's not that I *like* talking about the same thing but it's because self-care is important.

Learning to sleep, eat, exercise, communicate and not isolate keeps us sane. *Oh, and avoid alcohol and drugs!* Please! Learning how to do these things can be hard; it can feel impossible. It is, *yes,* exhausting.

I'm sick of the word *exhausted* right now but I believe it's important to *validate* why we often feel this way: to recognize that it's normal and will not always define our life. It's part of recovering from mental illness. It's part of the journey we take to find a place of stability. A place of, at the very least, relative peace." ---The Mighty

---

I saw my psychiatrist today like I do every month. I had some pretty bad anxiety, but it's over now. I asked my doctor what a reasonable expectation is for my recovery. He basically said it depends on the individual. His goal is to try and keep clients out of the hospital. If that can be achieved, then it's a baby steps approach to how much that person can handle. Some people can almost fully recover and live a "normal" life, and some clients can't. And it's a spectrum in between. He told me that there's no magic pill to make anyone feel better. He did say that he admired my strength and motivation. I believe that I have gotten better since I started seeing this doctor, so that's progress. I told him how frustrating mental illness can be because I can do the same thing for days or weeks, and get different results. He reminded me that mental illness is not logical like mathematics. That made me feel a little better for some reason. I'm always trying to find logical solutions to my symptoms, but sometimes, the symptoms cannot be avoided or explained. I plan on taking it easy the rest of the night.

I have to see the doctor today, which is always a bit rough, but I have a lot of positive progress to report. I'm not feeling the usual anxiety and panic that comes with my appointment. Two things my doctor told me that really helped me were "Do what makes you anxious" and "We're here to help you, not hurt you". No one in the psychiatric field wants to see you sick or fail. In the last couple months, I have been able to drive myself further distances, socialize, and lose weight among other things. Since I have so much experience with my illness (12+ years), I am able to better manage it. That means getting enough sleep, eating reasonably, thinking positively, staying sober, monitoring caffeine, taking my meds as scheduled, and avoiding triggers whenever I can. I got to the point where staying the same was more painful than taking the plunge and trying something differently. It's okay to fail, but try to think about "What if I succeed?". I was confined to my home for years, and I started taking chances. It's working. It's a little scary that my world is getting bigger, but it's better than being afraid to drive or socialize. I still have a lot of work to do, but there is no timetable on progress. You just have to do what you can, when you can. It has been extremely frustrating at times because I just wanted everything to be better instantly. Unfortunately, mental illness doesn't work that way. These were just a few thoughts and words of encouragement that I was thinking of right now. I hope it helps you in your journey.

Miracles don't always have to be supernatural like raising someone from the dead. Sometimes, it can be what doesn't happen to us or maybe something bad that happens to us that is a blessing in disguise. If I hadn't gotten treatment so long ago, who knows what could have happened to me. I could have gone to prison. I could have married the wrong person or had a child I couldn't care for. I could have died either by my own hand or excessive self-medication.

In this day, it has become cool not to care and to think that nothing really matters and that there's nothing out there greater than ourselves. But what if it all matters? What if everything is a divine plan that none of us can comprehend? Mind boggling, isn't it? And one last thing--- If you can't find a miracle, be the miracle.

I write about my mental health issues because it helps other people, and in turn, is therapeutic for me. I don't want to give the impression that my life is horrible. Not even close. I am truly blessed, and I try not to complain too much. Driving to downtown Cincinnati to the casino with my mom was a major victory. Losing 50 pounds (and hopefully more) is a major victory. Having a birthday party where I was social was a major victory. Today, a major victory is going to be getting in the shower and paying bills. Tomorrow, a major victory would be to go out and see some bands at a local bar. I wish I could tell you what I was working towards. I don't know if I will ever be fully functional, whatever that means. I would like to work for myself, but I have been looking into writing opportunities. My real dream since I was 19 years old is to be a professional poker player. I don't have the patience, and I get too anxious right now to be successful at that. I want to be able to drive myself to my own doctor appointments. I would like to be able to drive an hour to Dayton to visit my Alma Mater. I guess it's good to have some idea of what I want to accomplish. Anyways, the whole point is to let you know that my life is mostly good, all things considered. I write mainly about my struggles because mental illness rarely is talked about, especially from males. Not because I always struggle.

This might sound insensitive, but I have to get something off my chest. Life isn't easy or fair. Never has been, never will be. Complaining is poison. It's poison to yourself and everyone around you. If you don't like something about your life, you have to be willing to change something. Nothing will change if you don't change something. Treat yourself to something you like. Go for a drive. Meditate. Journal. Go on a rant like I am doing right now. It can be whatever brings you joy and relief. In a perfect world, everyone would choose healthy coping mechanisms, but sometimes it's excessive drinking, drugs, shopping, gambling, sex, or whatever other vices. I'm also guilty of all of this, but I think I do a good job of staying upbeat most of the time, all things considered. If you have food, shelter, clean drinking water, and clothing, you are blessed more than 25% of the entire world. If negative thoughts or a "woe is me" attitude enters your mind, think of 5 things to be grateful for or think 3 positive thoughts. I had to practice positivity and gratitude. It didn't just come to me. I had to work for it. Okay, rant over.

From November 2017:

I've had a couple of good weeks recently. I've been eating less, and controlling my coffee intake. Sleeping a little less during the day. I have even been smoking a little less because of the cold weather. I've been in a great mood. I had my little motivational note that I wrote to myself. Just trying to manage my symptoms. It kind of came to a halt today. In the afternoon, I was really anxious and my body was sore. I don't think that a lot of people realize all the symptoms that severe anxiety/panic can cause, like physical soreness. It felt like it was the most tired I have ever been in my life. I tried to eat a small meal and sleep it off. I'm trying to manage right now, and I thought I would feel better if I wrote about it. I didn't make it to my family's Thanksgiving dinner, and that's okay I guess. I kind of feel like I let my family down, but my family is pretty understanding. If you asked me why I couldn't go, it would be hard to explain. My anxiety is just there. It just is. I try to take my bad days and turn them into teaching moments for anyone who will listen. Some people will never "get it" or care, and that's fine. I can't convince everyone that mental illness is, in fact, an illness. It's not an improper mindset. It's a physical, brain disease. I share my life and struggles out of love, the greater good, and the sake of education.

I've been struggling with depression for a few weeks with little relief. Just general sadness, hopelessness, and irritability. I think I'm starting to come out of it, but the fight is leaving me exhausted. I have had some bursts of productive energy here and there, so that's good. I'm looking for direction right now in my life. I'm fortunate that I don't really have anything tying me down, so I have a lot of options except for my limitations on how much I can actually work and be productive. I'm fighting the good fight. I've always thought there was dignity in that. I want to be a good example to anyone dealing with hardships and similar issues.

It's good to have a short memory, never getting too high on success or too low with failure, but when I am in a dark place, I have to remember everything that I have accomplished. I always have a sense of urgency because I feel like I am living on borrowed time, and I don't take life for granted. Sometimes, this attitude leaves me frustrated because I don't feel like I am doing enough when I have to rest or when I have a bad day.

One of my favorite movies is "A Beautiful Mind". It's hard for me to watch now because of the main character's (Dr. John Nash played by Russell Crowe) struggle with mental illness. He was always looking for his magnum opus in the form of an original idea in terms of mathematics, whether it be a new formula or a solution to an old equation. I think I feel the same way, and I always felt a connection to Russell Crowe's character. I just want something to define my life that is all mine. So far, it has been my books and sharing my story. I'm not sure if I will ever eclipse this achievement, but I keep trying. I always joke around with my mom that I have already peaked and it's all downhill from here. Just joking, of course.

I put a lot of pressure on myself to go out and do things, but I think I'm just kind of a home body now. Large groups of people exhaust me, and it's not that I don't like people, I would just rather have a short visit with a few people. I prefer coffee over alcohol. I prefer quiet time over loudness. I prefer watching sports or reading over a night out. People change I think. I've had enough wild and exciting times to last a lifetime honestly, so maybe that's why I prefer more relaxing activities. Maybe I am getting old or maybe it's my illness, but either way, it doesn't matter. I shouldn't put unnecessary pressure on myself to go out if I feel like staying home.

I simply don't have the time or the energy to have hate in my heart or hold grudges. I have a ton of people who love me and need my help. I have very few enemies, and I don't know if that's a good thing or a bad thing, but I'll be damned if I'm going to let these people have a place in my heart. If someone fucks me over, they become irrelevant in my life. I don't wish harm on anyone. If karma doesn't do its job, then these people lost a good friend, and that's enough for me. Much love to the people who love me and support me.

I had to reschedule my doctor's appointment today, and my next appointment is after the first of the year. Maybe I can enjoy the holidays with my friends and family without having to worry about filling medications or attending appointments. The main reason I see a psychiatrist is so that he can refill my medications and make sure they are still working properly. I haven't changed medications in almost 8 years I think, maybe longer. He always asks the same questions, and we usually just end up talking about sports. I don't have a therapist or psychologist, but I have a case manager who basically plays that role and helps me if I have confusing paperwork.

I've shown a lot of progress with my anxiety and leaving the house, and I've also lost almost 60 pounds. I still have bad days, but I'm learning how to cope better every day. I do a lot of my own research to help deal with daily life. I work hard every day to get even better, and that's all I can ask of myself and hope for. I'm extremely hard on myself, but I'm working on letting a lot of stuff go.

The most dominant and frustrating symptom that I am dealing with right now is physical exhaustion. I can barely stay awake. I have body soreness almost everywhere as well. I have lost weight (almost 60 pounds), and I drink coffee to try and help, but most of the time, I am tired. If I drink too much coffee, I have a panic attack. It's a delicate balance, and I treat coffee just like medication. I have to be very careful. I have a hard time sleeping at night, so I have to take naps during the day. It's been like this for years. Today was a pretty good day besides spilling coffee everywhere haha. I took out the trash, unloaded the dishwasher, addressed a computer problem, and took a shower. Tasks like these that are simple to most, are difficult for me. Most days are pretty good, but of course I still have bad days. There are days when I feel like a burden and a failure. There are days when I really don't accomplish anything worth noting. On good days, I feel like a success and an asset to my family and friends. This is bipolar disorder. Two polar opposites. I try to stay somewhere in the middle, but this is a strong, serious illness. On bad days, I try to practice positive thinking and gratitude to offset the negative thoughts and depression. I try to treat myself and have things to look forward to. I remind myself of everything I have accomplished. It's a flat out war every single day.

The only reason I would ever want a lot of money is to be generous with it. Luxury is nice, but it doesn't buy what my heart is after. I just want to help and inspire people without having to worry about my mental health everyday. Money can't buy that. Money can't buy a lot of things that I want. I've pretty much accepted the fact that I'm going to have to deal with my mental health every day. It's just frustrating. It's not like I want to do something outrageous with my life, like buy mansions and yachts or something. I like being "the man", and I used to be to a lot of people. I dream about passing out $100 bills to the poor and my friends. I love buying drinks for everyone at the bar. Buying 100 double cheeseburgers to pass out to the hungry and homeless. Stuff like that. I swear that I would volunteer at a soup kitchen or something similar if I had the energy. At least I have my books and my mental health page that I work on. That's enough feeling sorry for myself.

I'm actually pretty proud of myself. My truck wouldn't start, so I called AAA. They sent a guy out to test my battery and alternator. My battery needs to be replaced, which will be an expense, but my alternator is still in really good shape. That's good news. More good news is that my truck was in the driveway when it wouldn't start instead of out and about. I handled all of this with extreme calm and maturity. I know that might not sound like much to most of you, but it's an accomplishment for me.

There was a football coach named Greg Schiano who used to say (paraphrasing here), "If you find yourself in a forest, start chopping wood". In this metaphor, if you are surrounded by tall trees, it's not going to help to stand there. You have to start chopping wood. DO SOMETHING. No matter what you are battling, you have to start somewhere. It's an active decision. If you don't like something about your life, you have to make an active decision to change something. Start infinitesimally small if you have to. For me, small things that I do to get out of a funk are: taking a shower, taking a drive, cleaning up after myself, journaling, reading, listening to music, and just generally anything that is difficult for me to do. Afterward, I feel accomplished and better about myself that I at least tried.

I think the goal of my medication and treatment is to keep me somewhere "in the middle" as far as mood and behavior goes. For someone with bipolar one, there's nothing worse. My spirit just wants to be "up" and happy all the time. I try to circumvent the system by drinking coffee. This usually jolts me into hypomania (a lesser version of full mania), and at it's worst, a panic attack. I'm not only fighting bipolar one with psychotic features, I am also battling anxiety and panic attacks. Other things can trigger mania also. Usually when something good happens or goes my way or I get excited for whatever reason. I know it's probably a weird concept to think that being too happy is a bad thing, but it is for someone with my brand of bipolar disorder. I am more manic than depressed, which is why I have bipolar one instead of bipolar two. Bipolar two is more depressed than manic, but both brands have features of both. I have been mostly depressed for a few months, but I always have bouts of mania sprinkled in. Bipolar depression is physically painful (body soreness), and can lead to sleep disturbances, suicidal idealization (thoughts), excessive crying, weight gain or weight loss, and poor diet and hygiene.

Bipolar disorder is an illness of extremes. Really high highs and really low lows. These manic and depressed episodes can last hours, days, weeks, or years. It all depends on the person. I feel like I am coming out of my depressed mood, but I never know how long any mood is going to last. I think that's why my doctor tries to keep me in the middle, like I mentioned earlier. There's so much more to all of this, which is why I write about it whenever I can.

"What you take for granted, someone is praying for". I try to remember this when times are hard, but I hope all of you with healthy brains learn something from me and all my posts about my illness. I had a great day. A great day for me means: taking a shower\personal hygiene, running an errand with no driving anxiety, cooking lunch, changing my clothes, and taking out the trash. Most of you do these things every day with no problems. Just know that there are so many people fighting battles that thankfully, you will never know anything about. I have a grateful heart, but my life is hard sometimes. I know there are so many people who have it harder, but it doesn't help to hear that when I'm struggling. I think everyone can relate to that. I try not to complain and I am blessed in many ways, but surviving mental illness is the toughest thing I've ever had to do.

You are going to come across people in your life who are always critical, negative, and see no issue in their own flaws, if they even believe that they have flaws. Some of us seek approval from these people, and we drive ourselves crazy trying to get this approval. It's frustrating, but no matter what you do, you are never going to get that approval and reassurance from these kinds of people. I could quit smoking, lose 300 pounds, write 10 more books, and become President, and there will still be people that I cannot please. Give your love, energy, and attention to supportive people who are going to build you up, not see you for your flaws. I know that personally, I need to hear that I am doing a good job every so often. A lot of people are like that, but not everyone. I think people with mental illness are especially sensitive and need reassurance more than the general population. It's hard to believe that I am doing the right thing when progress sometimes seems stagnant or slow. When all I can do one day is take a shower, it's hard to believe that I am doing a good job. When you can't find anyone to support you, you just have to believe it in your heart. If you are doing the best you can, that is literally all you can do.

One thing that irritates me is when older people tell me I am too young to worry about certain things, especially death. For one, worrying about death is a clinical symptom of my illness. For another, I have felt like I was going to die so many times, whether it be from a panic attack or otherwise, that I have learned my lesson as far as wasting time goes. I hate being in a bad mood because I feel like I am wasting valuable time. Being in a bad mood sometimes is also part of my illness, so you can see the problem there. For some reason, when you are mentally ill or disabled, people stop thinking that your time is valuable. I just argued that my time is actually more valuable, at least to me. I don't mind wasting time on fun things or things that I enjoy. Sometimes, I give myself a hard time when I can't get out of a depressed or irritable mood. Part of that is because I feel like I am wasting time, but another part is that for someone with bipolar one, being in a bad mood is one of the worst places to be.

January 24, 2019

I had some small victories yesterday. I had an appointment to do some market research. I drove myself, and I earned a little money. Market research is when companies pay people like me for my opinion on a wide range of things from coffee to disposable razor blades. It's hard to qualify sometimes, but it's nice to earn a little extra money. I have been doing market research for years. Showing up to do the survey at a certain time is hard for me too because I have anticipatory anxiety, which means I get anxiety when I anticipate having to be somewhere at a certain time. I think it can also mean that I anticipate on having anxiety when I get there. I had a little anxiety, but the appointment only lasted about an hour total, including driving time. Another thing I accomplished was that I unloaded the dishwasher. I know that doesn't sound like much, but it's hard for me because I am constantly sore and exhausted, so it's hard to get motivation to do small tasks like this.

January 24, 2019

I kind of figured it was going to happen, but I wanted to believe that maybe I would escape my progress unharmed. This morning, I felt completely awful. I was in so much pain from anxiety that all I could do is lay in my bed until the pain went away enough for me to sleep it off. I don't know if it's because I hadn't gotten enough sleep or if I overdid it with my daily activities and responsibilities. It always happens, but these awful feelings have gotten less intense and less frequent over time. I honestly felt like I might die or need to go to the hospital. Whether that is accurate medically or not is irrelevant. The feelings are real to me. I just wanted to say how much love I have for many of you, even if we have never met or hung out. I'm so grateful it's over that I wanted to write something of substance and let everyone know that I still have love in my heart.

January 26, 2019

I took a shower tonight, which has been difficult for me since I was hospitalized and diagnosed. Mental illness and its medications are exhausting plus I am a large person, so there's a physical element to showers as well. For me, it's more my illness that makes showers difficult. I get claustrophobic in the shower, and I have bad memories from the tiny community showers in the hospital all the way back in 2006. Back then, I remember having to earn the trust of the nurses to use a razor for my face. I guess they wanted to make sure that I wouldn't use it on myself or anyone else. Understandable I guess. Something so simple as a shower can be an ordeal. I don't think most people think of little tasks like this when they think of mental illness. That's why I think this book and my experiences are so important to the understanding of mental illness.

January 27, 2019

This is something I really struggle with. I have a very strong guilt complex. I feel guilty for resting sometimes when I am weak, and I feel guilty for putting my family through everything regarding my mental illness in the last 13 years. I also feel guilty about how I treated my parents when I was younger. I was very rebellious, and I got into drinking and drugs. I heard something one time that I am trying to embrace that states, "Forgive yourself for things when you didn't know any better". I'm not really sure that describes my situation, but it does apply to some events in my life. I knew that drinking and drugs were the wrong thing to do, but I guess I just didn't care. I guess I thought I was invincible. I could probably argue that a lot of teenagers and young adults go through this, but I didn't have the same heart back then. My parents are both close to 80 years old, and I worry so much about them. I love them with all my heart, and I was rude, selfish, and careless all those years ago. Even though I made a lot of mistakes, I have to find a way to forgive myself in order to move forward, and I recommend that you find a way to forgive yourself as well.

January 28, 2019

I can only speak for myself, and I don't claim to know everything, but happiness doesn't lie in money and possessions. I know money helps because that's what the world runs on, but at the end of the day, it can't buy happiness. From my own personal experiences, I feel the most happy and satisfied when I feel like my life has a purpose. When I do good for others. When I'm a loyal, honest friend. When I have a good day as far as my symptoms go. Things like that. Money can't buy satisfaction with your life. I've had a lot of money before and I've been broke, but I learned that I can be happy in either situation and all situations in between. People spend their whole lives chasing dollars, but that's not where it's at. Money may cure some of my problems, but it can't cure my illness, and it can't buy the health of my loved ones.

January 30, 2019

I have repetitive thoughts pretty often. The thoughts can be song lyrics, simple tasks that are on my mind, or practicing in my mind what I am going to speak out loud. Song lyrics can be especially frustrating because sometimes the same song will be stuck in my head for weeks. It starts as soon as a wake up, and I have to find a way to divert my attention for it to stop. If I have a task or obligation to complete, I will think about it over and over until it is finished. I am a confident speaker, but I catch myself repeating in my head what I am going to say. When it's really bad, I have repetitive, negative thoughts. These thoughts are usually about death, whether it be mine or a loved one's.

February 1, 2019

Managing money can be difficult for someone with bipolar disorder. It is definitely true for me. I get my disability payment anywhere from the first to the third of the month, depending on business days falling on weekends. It's usually the third of the month, but this month, the third falls on a Sunday, so I received my payment today (Friday). Something strange happens to me when I get paid. I shouldn't say strange. I know what it is. It's mania. I get so ramped up, and I just want to spend all my money in a day. Disability is supposed to last for the whole month, and I usually don't save enough to make it through until the end of the month. It's so frustrating because I know myself by now, and I know the mania is coming, but it's so hard to fight. Mania and spending money gives me such a high. It doesn't help that I'm usually broke, so when I have money, it's almost foreign territory. I have had spending problems for years. If I ever receive a large sum of money, I am thinking about letting one of my relatives control the funds. I think that's the responsible thing to do, even though it makes me feel inadequate and childish.

February 1, 2019

I don't leave the house very often. It's probably because of my anxiety, but I have also lost interest in a lot of activities outside the house. However, there are rare occasions when I force myself to do things that involve driving myself and leaving the house, whether in a social setting or by myself. It's such a great feeling of accomplishment when I push through my anxiety and depression and have a good time. My body and mind are telling me "No, you can't do that", but I push through it regardless and usually have a good time. That feeling of accomplishment when I get home, exhausted, and lay in bed knowing that I did the best I could in those moments. That despite my mind and body being uncooperative, I succeeded in beating my anxiety and depression. My doctor told me one time, "Do what makes you anxious", and honestly, I looked at him like he was the one who needed help, but it's true. With every little successful step, things that once made me anxious get easier.

Taking a shower is a perfect example. I take more showers now than I have in recent years. I used to get dizzy and have flashbacks. I just kept trying, and now, taking a shower isn't even really a big accomplishment for me. It's a little sad and disheartening because taking a shower used to be a huge accomplishment for me. If I took a shower in a day, I could rest the remainder of the day and feel satisfied. Taking a shower doesn't satisfy my need to succeed anymore. At least not to the highest degree like it used to.

There's no magic pill for many ailments, and sometimes I have to force myself outside my comfort zone, as uncomfortable at first as it may be.

February 3, 2019

It's my beloved mom's birthday today. She is the glue that holds the household together. She is so caring, kind, and selfless. I will never regret spending so much time with my mom and dad. Many people don't have their parents left here on Earth, and I know I am lucky to be in my situation.

Unrelated, but I had a weight loss victory today. I bought a pair of shoes about 5 years ago that cost me about $100. They aren't anything special. It's just that gym shoes in men's size 15 cost that much. I only wore them a few times back then, and then I gained so much weight that my feet and ankles swelled so that I couldn't wear these nice shoes anymore. I took them out of my closet last night, and they fit! I was very pleased, and it's one of those amazing things that come with weight loss.

February 4, 2019

Every so often, if the feeling gets me, I like to thank my friends and family for loving and supporting me through my mental illness journey. The easiest way for me to reach the most people is through social media. So, thank you for loving me and supporting me when my mental and physical health was most in question. People probably think I am crazier than I actually am clinically because I am very vocal about telling people I love them and I care. That's one positive takeaway I've had through all of this. Life is short, unpredictable, and not guaranteed to anyone. I go to bed at night with little regret and a satisfaction of knowing that I told people how I feel.

Another positive takeaway was that I found my purpose in life, at least for the time being. It's been about 7 years since I decided to become a mental health advocate, and eventually write 2 books, with a third one (this book) on the way. Maybe one day my purpose and mission will change, but for now, being an advocate has brought me satisfaction with my life that I never could have imagined.

February 6, 2019

I saw something the other day referring to mental illness that read, "Of course it's all in my head. That's where my brain is." I really wish mental illness could be renamed "brain illness" or "brain disorder". Something to incorporate the term brain to let others know that mental illness is a dysfunction of an actual organ and it's not "all in your head", so to speak. If someone breaks an arm, everyone rushes to help and sign the cast. A broken arm is visible and tangible. People can relate to that. When you have mental illness, which is invisible, except for the outward symptoms, it's hard for most people to grasp the concept. It's not their fault. It's just human nature to have an easier time believing in something you can touch and feel. Mental illness is mysterious in that way. You can have 100 people with the same disorder, but the severity ranges, the symptoms are similar, but the experience is unique to each individual.

February 7, 2019

I'm not a big fan of the baby steps approach to doing things, but it works for a lot of people. I am an all or nothing kind of person. It could be my bipolar disorder or my personality or both. I've had so many days where I told myself, "If you can just take a shower for the day, you are a success." I'm struggling a little bit today, and I want to take a shower after I'm done writing this. To be fair with myself, I have been working very hard lately and making some progress. It's always at a slower pace than I would prefer, but progress nonetheless.

Getting out of a rut from depression and anxiety can start with a task as small as taking a shower. Anything you can do to give yourself hope that things can change, do it. Get some fresh air. Put on fresh clothes. Treat yourself to some ice cream or whatever you enjoy doing. If you see a ray of sunshine peek through the clouds, grab onto it and don't let go. Hope is depression and anxiety's enemy, and hope can be hard to come by. I understand feeling hopeless, when it feels like everything is such a chore. I'm not totally opposed to just riding out the depression, but things usually don't change on their own, and at some point, you have to reach down deep and just try to help yourself. When you are depressed and anxious and in a rut, what do you have to lose?

February 8, 2019

I don't hate anyone or wish harm on anyone. If I don't like someone, I just simply cut them out of my life. I would think this would be a good way to act, and maybe that's why I was spared. I don't really know how other people go about their lives. I don't have the time or energy to waste on people who don't like me. There's so many people in my life that love me that deserve my love in return. I don't know if I believe in karma exactly, but at some point, I do believe you reap what you sow. I doubt karma because I see plenty of good things happen to bad people and vice versa. For me, to live a happy fulfilling life, I need to simplify a lot of things about my life, and holding grudges and hating people is just one of those things that doesn't have a place.

Of course, by nature, 1 get in bad moods. I can be mean spirited too, but I like to believe that I always apologize if I feel I was wrong. I don't really argue a lot with people either. It seems like arguing has become somewhat of a fad or trendy in recent times. It's the time and energy and simplification of life thing again. I firmly believe that are people who actually enjoy arguing and stirring the pot just because, and I really don't understand those types of people.

February 10, 2019

It's Sunday. I had a pretty bad day yesterday. I was in a generally crabby mood and completely exhausted. I feel asleep several times with a coffee cup in my hand. I just couldn't get up the energy to do much of anything. I always feel like I wasted the weekend when I don't leave the house. I am 37 years old now, and it seems like people my age are either doing the family thing, or they drink alcohol all weekend. I wish I got joy out of going out to eat or going to the movies or similar activities. I wonder whether it's my personality, or if it's just easier to stay home because of my anxiety and depression symptoms. I am quickly bored and can barely sit still sometimes, so I don't have a lot of patience either. I hate that I am that way, but it's all part of the package. I get extremely upset if I am hungry and have to wait even the smallest length of time for food. It just makes me anxious to have to wait for pretty much anything, so I think I just avoid a lot of things to save the aggravation. I know that's not the mentally healthiest thing to do, but it saves me a lot of frustration. Maybe one of these days I will try to go out to eat or go to a movie just to see what happens and how I react. I guess a panic attack and aggravation are the worst things that can happen. It has to be better than feeling trapped in my house.

February 11, 2019

Bipolar disorder and anxiety are two disorders that tend to run together. Disorders that come in pairs or groups are said to be co-morbid, or co-morbidity. This is true in my diagnosis. I have told you my complete diagnosis, but mania, depression, and anxiety are the strongest symptoms that I face. There's something called the vicious cycle of anxiety. When I first wake up for the day or from a daily nap, I can't stand being tired, so I drink coffee. I always make sure the coffee is near a medication time. When I finally get up the energy to be productive, I might buzz around for a bit, but eventually I take my medication and usually eat a meal and go back to sleep. I have been fighting this cycle for at least 7 years, and that's just how far back I can remember. My memory is hit or miss these days. It's a delicate balance, and really I'm playing with fire as I have given myself panic attacks many times. Trying to be energized but calm has been a daily battle for a very long time. Being lethargic is such a horrible feeling for me. I don't have the energy to be productive in the slightest. Plus, people with bipolar one tend to want to be "up" all the time (mania), which I have to monitor so that I avoid skipping sleep or making bad decisions. I was manic for so many years that I just thought that's how life was meant to be. That's what hard workers did. I am still adjusting almost 13 years later on how to rest and make sure I get enough sleep.

One thing that is somewhat rare about me is that I have only missed one dose of medication in those 13 years. I have been compliant, which really isn't my nature, but it probably saved my life. Sometimes, medications make people feel better so they stop taking them, which almost always leads to a downward spiral, and it's back to a condition at least as bad before the medications were initiated.

February 12, 2019

I live with my parents in a house that they have lived in since 1967, four years after they were married. It's the only place that has ever felt like home to me. My ego is a little bruised because I have to live with them, being 37 years old. My parents are very supportive and understanding, as much as they can. They know that social and family functions are hard for me, and they don't expect me to come, but they always let me know I'm invited. My parents help me with anything from paying my bills to cleaning, house chores, and laundry. They are both close to 80 years old, and I know it's a great time to hang around them. I help out around the house whenever I can, but they really don't pressure me to do a lot around the house.

I don't know if anyone can truly understand mental illness unless they have it, but my parents do a pretty remarkable job. After all, they have 13 years of experience with my abilities, symptoms, and personality as well. I love them with all my heart, and we have a pretty good relationship. Support is so crucial to recovery success, and I am blessed to have a lot, whether it's from my parents, siblings, other family, or close friends. I try to be that support for others who might not have the support that I have, as a way of paying it forward.

February 13, 2019

The first thing I was diagnosed with in 2006 was bipolar disorder with psychotic features. I have bipolar one, which means I experience more mania than depression. Bipolar two is the opposite. Manic and depressive episodes vary in length. They can last hours, days, weeks, months, or even years. The reason I bring this diagnosis up is so that I can talk about the psychotic features part of this diagnosis. Psychosis is a total break from reality. I think it's what most people think of when they hear "crazy", just to put it simply. I haven't been in a psychotic episode for many years, but it was like watching myself in a movie, and I was the star of the show. I had no control over what my mind was telling me to do. My doctor always asks if I hear voices, and I always say no, because I feel like the "voices" in my head are just my inner dialogue. I think everyone has an inner dialogue. It's when the voices become directive that it's a problem, meaning the voices are actually telling you to do something or you feel compelled to do something with no control.

I don't know if it's psychosis or not, but sometimes I can feel my thoughts accelerate and become jumbled. I don't know how else to describe it as that it feels like I'm losing touch with reality. These episodes happen when I am manic or anxious. The feeling of going crazy is a symptom of anxiety and panic, so that's what I usually chalk it up to. These mini-psychotic episodes also happen when I haven't been getting the proper amount of sleep, or if I drink too much coffee, or both.

I definitely have respect for these disorders and what they can do. I am very careful to get enough sleep (when I can), and use my best judgment when drinking coffee, which is very frequently, or alcohol, which is very rare for me. I really think about what I put into my body. I used to self-medicate every day with alcohol and marijuana, but now, I prefer the feeling of being in control as much as possible. To be honest, if alcohol and marijuana still made me feel good, I would still do it. Somewhere along the way, the calming effects and fun that I had went away. I know I am better off, but I miss those days. I had a lot of fun.

February 15, 2019

I have no idea how long I had been psychotic before I was hospitalized in 2006. It seems like it was a week or two, but I was also manic, so I was making poor decisions too. One thing I remember about psychosis is that I thought that ordinary things like TV commercials, songs, and lottery tickets had secret messages in them for me to discover. I thought these messages were leading me to a gift from the CIA, for whom I thought I was working for. I opened a stranger's car door and sat in the driver's seat because I thought it was a gift from the CIA. I remember thinking about starting up the car. Thank God no one left the keys in the ignition. I was arrested for trespassing and criminal damaging. The charges were dropped by a not guilty by reason of insanity defense.

I thought there were CIA agents on my roof, and I remember thinking that there were hidden microphones in my house. One of these messages landed me at my parents' house, and that's when my family noticed something was wrong. My brother, who is like a second father to me, told me to lay down on my bed until I calmed down. Then, he convinced me to take a ride with him. I didn't know where we were going, but thank God I trusted him. We were going to the hospital. My first admission date was July 31, 2006. I was in the hospital locked down like a prisoner until August 11 of that year. As you could imagine, this whole experience changed me and was necessary to start recovering.

February 16, 2019

I've been overweight my whole life. When I was a kid, I had trouble fitting into the desks at school. I had trouble fitting into sports uniforms. Basically anything where sizing was involved, I had trouble fitting into whatever it was. Even when I was in tip-top shape playing football in high school, I was 313 pounds. I am also over 6 feet tall. Being overweight isn't a crime. What I'm really getting at is that there are a lot of businesses and establishments that don't have seating that an overweight person can fit in. For example, a restaurant where there are only booths and the tables don't move. Any chairs with "arms" on them. If overweight people want to buy clothes, they usually cost extra and aren't as fashionable. Not to mention the sizing for me in a T-shirt is XXXXL, at least, and makes you feel like some humongous monster. It really is a form of discrimination. I don't understand why people don't speak up more. High top tables are horrible too because the chairs usually have smaller seats and they are elevated with a less than sturdy base to hold the person's weight. It's not comfortable to try and balance and defy gravity while I am trying to enjoy a meal or beer. All I am proposing is that businesses dedicate a portion of their seating to bigger folks so that overweight people can enjoy what smaller people get to enjoy. Being overweight isn't a punishable offense. I have lost over 60 pounds now, but no matter how much weight I lose, I will never be skinny. I'm cool with that. I actually kind of like being big because it intimidates people into not starting fights with me or harassing me in some other capacity.

I also excelled at sports because I was bigger than all the other kids. As someone who is overweight with anxiety, I have to worry about every place I go whether that business will have accommodating seating. I wanted to write about this because no one ever talks about it, and it's a major issue for overweight people.

February 18, 2019

I have been receiving disability payments for about 3 years now. I got sick in 2006, and it took me 7 years of hard fighting to get approved. I don't understand how the process works because I felt like I had a strong case. I tried to return to work several times, and each time, it resulted in a nervous breakdown, sometimes requiring hospitalization. I also have insurance for my psychiatric visits and medications. I have started to feel better in general in the last couple of weeks, so I have been looking for small jobs that I might be able to do. My friend gave me an Ebay project to sort through a sports collectibles collection to see if I could find anything of value, and I would get half of the sales. That's what I'm currently working on besides this book and my mental health page on social media. It used to be that I couldn't even think or talk about a job without getting extremely anxious and upset.

I was standing in line at the gas station the other day and I had a flashback-type memory. I remembered how hard it used to be for me to drive myself less than a mile up the street, and then interact with a cashier, for example. I used to get dizzy and chest pains when I had to be social at all. I had a hard time making and keeping eye contact too. I think it's because my confidence was destroyed. I lost my confidence when I couldn't leave the house at all, be social, or make eye contact. You just don't feel good about yourself.

February 18, 2019

Success and recovery can be a scary thing for someone with mental illness. You might ask yourself 'why?'...Well, with recovery and wellness come higher expectations, and what if I or that person can't live up to them? What if I fail? What if I have a relapse? These are typical thoughts when someone who is ill has a string of time when things are going well. Good days are what I fight and pray for, but I am always skeptical and cautious. You can think of that as a sad thing, or I think of it as monitoring my illness. I know that if I start feeling a little too happy and I don't sleep as much, that could be a sign of a manic episode coming. I think the best defense to prevent a manic episode from getting out of control is awareness and acknowledgment of it and sleep.

If I am feeling sad for no reason and sleeping a lot, I know those are signs of a depressive episode, and I need to do whatever I can to get out of it. I need to treat myself, or take a walk, or get some air. Sometimes, it seems like nothing helps, and I feel like I just have to sleep and tough it out. My medications are designed to keep me somewhere in the middle, and they do a pretty good job of that for the most part. I have changed medications several times in the last 13 years, but I have been on the same combination for several years with no major emergencies. I take Invega and Trileptal for my mood. They are also anti-psychotics. I take Klonopin for anxiety, as needed. So, with all my troubles, I am only on 3 medications. I don't think it's something to be proud of exactly, but I have friends who really struggle and take over 40 pills a day.

February 19, 2019

I think my sense of humor has helped me greatly in coping with mental illness. I enjoy making people laugh, and it helps me have a light heart about it all as well. When I was released from the hospital in 2006, I was joking just days into my recovery. I don't exactly remember what I joked about way back when, but I do know that I had been incapacitated for days, which turned into years (I think). All I could do was eat, sleep, and go to the bathroom. Taking a shower wasn't even close to being an option. Sometimes, I feel like I am almost addicted to cracking jokes, but I suppose there are worse things. I am on social media a lot cracking jokes, and I think that people take me more seriously in a way when I am serious.

When I'm not joking around, I am advocating for the mentally ill and trying to help people understand who may be interested. Mental illness is so common that it would be hard to believe too many people who haven't been affected by it; whether it be themselves, a relative, or a friend. I try to set a good example and stay positive for all my loved ones. I never want anyone to give me pity. My friends and family are there for me when I need someone to just listen. Lots of people think that when someone like myself vents that I am looking for advice. I am almost never looking for advice. Sometimes, I just need a listening ear and an understanding heart.

February 20, 2019

Freshmen year of college was the only year from about age 15 until my diagnosis that I didn't have a traditional job. I think all freshmen at the University of Dayton were required to live in the dorms. It was a pretty great set up. I had a university card that paid for my meals, and my parents would load money on it every so often if I wanted to eat from a restaurant instead of the university cafeterias. I also tried to work after my diagnosis, but the employment always ended in a nervous breakdown or hospitalization. Ironically, freshmen year was the year that I had my lowest GPA. Life was easy back then. All I had to worry about was school, and I continued the pattern of self-medicating with alcohol and marijuana from high school.

After freshmen year, to save money, I got an apartment off campus and secured a job as a pizza delivery driver. I was working at my job up to 60 hours a week and trying to handle school work at the same time. At some point, a girl moved in with me and we dated for a few years. Juggling all of these things was probably when I was most manic, but it's hard to really pinpoint when it all started. Maybe even as early as childhood. I know I wasn't sleeping much, and I was self-medicating with alcohol and marijuana. Self-medicating was every day. I rarely got a day off of either work or school, and if I did get time off, I still wouldn't sleep. I continued like this for years. It came to a boiling point when I was first hospitalized in July-August of 2006. I still have manic episodes, but they are to a lesser degree and less frequent. I also have depressive episodes, but they are few and far between.

One thing that is very important to me as someone with bipolar disorder is something called sleep discipline. All it means is that I am extremely aware of how much sleep I am getting. I don't have a traditional sleep schedule, but I make sure that I sleep "enough" hours. It's not an exact number, and it hinges on my mood and energy. I have to take naps during the day to account for the sleep I miss during nightly hours. Lack of sleep can be a warning sign that might trigger a manic episode. I would definitely rather sleep too much than not much at all.

Sleeping can be an escape for me, from symptoms and life in general, assuming I can lay still long enough to actually fall asleep. In order to help my brain shut down, sometimes I have to turn off every light including the TV just so I have complete darkness and silence. That seems to help me focus on relaxing and drifting into sleep. Other times, I just relax my mind and body even if I can't sleep.

February 21, 2019

I talked to a friend of mine last night who struggles with anxiety and depression. She recently sought treatment for these conditions. She had been treated before, but it either got worse, or her medicine stopped working. She told me I was an inspiration, and she thanked me for always caring about her and checking in with her. We've always just been friends. Ever since grade school actually. It's always great to hear praise of course. I try to be an inspiration and a worthy advocate, but honestly, even I get sick of talking about mental illness sometimes. I just figure it needs to be done, and it's for the greater good. When I don't feel very inspirational, I simply don't have the positive energy to educate and advocate, and I'm not much of a help to anyone. This doesn't happen very often, but mental illness is such a big part of my life, and then to write about it constantly can be burdensome. I usually just wait until my negative feelings pass, and they always do eventually. I will take a break from writing and social media if I feel I need it. That is a very rare thing for me to do, but sometimes, it must be done for my own mental health.

February 22, 2019

Yesterday, I had lunch with one of my older brothers. The same brother who convinced me to take a ride to the hospital back in 2006. He was in high school when I was born, and he used to take me around and show me off to his friends. We have always been close, and he is like a second father to me. We just went to a fast food restaurant, but I had to drive myself there, sit still for an extended period of time, make eye contact, and have conversations with strangers. All of these things are challenges for me and have been for years. I would like to think I am getting better at these challenges, but I am always skeptical and always grateful when I can overcome these obstacles. My illness will probably never earn my trust, per se. I am always on the defensive because I don't like setbacks and I know how powerful my disorders are. I've seen what they can do to me.

February 25, 2019

One day at a time. One task at a time. One breath at a time. One step at a time. I repeat these things to myself sometimes when my mind is racing and my thoughts are jumbled. I try to take deep breaths and repeat this sort of mantra to myself to calm myself down. It helps to think as every little thing as a challenge where I can rest after I am finished. Resting after a task and the feeling of satisfaction is its own reward. Sometimes, it's simply taking a shower and putting on clean clothes, and other days, the tasks might be more challenging like seeing the doctor.

I have to see a nurse practitioner in two days because my usual doctor has left the clinic. I am always nervous to make the 20 minute drive to the clinic, but I am a little extra anxious because it's a new person. Who knows, this may be just another step in my progress, and maybe this guy will be an awesome person. I think I have made enough progress that I may only have to go to the clinic every 2-3 months, instead of every month. I can't remember the last time I saw the doctor, but I have had an extended break, and I have been much happier. When I have to see the doctor every month, I don't feel like a free person. I spend 3 weeks out of the month worrying about the appointment, so it's like my brain never really gets relief. My symptoms, like not being able to drive often, already make me feel like a prisoner in my own home. Every limitation I have makes me upset, and I always think back to the times when I didn't have to deal with mental illness. In a lot of ways, my life is better and definitely safer, after my diagnosis and treatment, but I also had a lot of fun when I was younger and more carefree. That's probably how it goes for a lot of people.

February 26, 2019

It's Tuesday night around 10 P.M. I have to see a nurse practitioner tomorrow at 2 P.M. I had the same doctor for many years, but he left the clinic I belong to. I honestly don't know the difference between a doctor and a nurse practitioner. I'm guessing several years of schooling. Hopefully, the NP will be a nice person, and this will be the beginning of a good relationship and more progress. I'm not very nervous about the appointment right now, but my anxiety will probably get worse as the appointment time approaches.

There are lots of really sick people at the clinic I go to for treatment. It's traumatic for me because the environment reminds me of being in the hospital. It's hard seeing so many mentally ill people together, and it's hard for me to talk about my symptoms. It's much easier for me to write about them. Even leaving the house for an extended amount of time is hard for me right now, but I feel like I have been making progress in the last year or so. Little by little, I have been able to do more things outside the house. I have been seeing my former doctor once a month for many years, and I'm hoping I will only have to see the NP every 2-3 months. I think I do better with a more hands off approach, and any time I can avoid the clinic, it's a good thing for my stress levels. My anxiety prevents me from leaving the house much, but I always have trouble finding things to do anyway. I bore very easily, and activities like going to a movie or out to dinner are stressful for me mainly because I have to sit still for long periods of time. I don't like feeling confined to a certain area or forced to stay still. I get very antsy, and my muscles get stiff. Sitting still is just all around uncomfortable for me, but there are times when it is much easier for me to do. There are other times when sitting still is near impossible, and I pace around the house or go in and out of the front door to get fresh air. When I feel antsy like that, I usually try to write or have a cigarette or two to calm down. I also roll my own cigarettes, and that activity is boring and keeps my hands busy even if my mind and body are overly active. I also do breathing exercises and grounding, which is basically making mental notes of my surroundings of things that I can use my five senses on. Grounding helps me feel in the moment, and not so much out of my mind and body. This out of body feeling is called disassociation I believe. I experience this quite often, but sometimes it's my own fault for drinking too much caffeine. I think a lot of people feel weird if they drink too much coffee, but I really have to watch it. If I drink too much, I can elicit a panic attack or mania. I pretty much have my dosage of coffee down to a science by now, but every once in a while, the caffeine will surprise me and send me into a panic attack or mild mania.

February 27, 2019

Whether you have a mental illness or not, I think a lot of people reach a point in their life, call it a rut, where staying the same hurts more than to change. At some point, you have to try something new for happiness and self-preservation. I feel like I am approaching that point nearer and nearer every day. I am starting to push myself a little more and venture out of my comfort zone because the days were running together and I was extremely depressed and frustrated. I hope you reach that point where you are well enough and brave enough to push yourself for a better life. Same goes for those without a mental illness. What's better than being happy and satisfied with your life? I haven't found anything better yet. I understand that depression, anxiety, bipolar symptoms, and other mental illnesses are completely overwhelming at times. I've had depression so severe that I couldn't get off the couch for months, possibly longer. I've had anxiety and panic so severe that I couldn't move or speak and I thought I was having a heart attack. It seemed like every week I was calling the hospital. When symptoms are this severe, it's not a matter of will. There is definitely something chemically wrong in the brain, and the most we can hope for is a medication or other treatment to help bring us out of it. But when you start to feel a little better, be brave enough to push yourself and try new things. It's extremely uncomfortable sometimes, but it's worth a better life for you.

I get great satisfaction from overcoming obstacles. If I do something that is very difficult for me, I usually have to rest in bed for a short time, but it's a great feeling of accomplishment. When I feel like I am making progress, my mood and attitude improves. I don't feel like such a prisoner in my own mind and in my own home. I feel normal, even though there is no such thing. It's one thing to have limitations, but when you internalize the limitations, and start getting on your own case, it can be very disheartening and depressing.

February 28, 2019

Yesterday, I had to go to the clinic and meet my new doctor. He's a young guy and seemed very nice. I felt comfortable talking to him, and he kept using words like "bro" and "dude", which I thought was funny. I lost another 2 pounds for a total of 62 pounds lost, and my blood pressure went down. The nurse practitioner, who I am just going to refer to as my doctor, kept me on the same medications. I have reached a point where I only have to see him every 3 months, instead of every month, which I had been doing for years. The doctor is not thrilled that I am on an anti-anxiety medication called Klonopin, but my track record has been successful and non-addicting, so he allowed me to continue taking it. The reason the doctor is concerned is because medications like Klonopin, "Benzos" for short, can cause early onset dementia. I would rather have relief from anxiety now and worry about getting old when I get there. Going to the clinic used to cause me so much stress, anxiety, and trauma that I would have to recover, mainly by sleeping, for at least a week. I felt really good yesterday, but I am having trouble recovering, which I did not anticipate. I have fallen asleep several times with coffee in my hand. I am trying my best to get my energy back that I had before my doctor's appointment. It will come back eventually, but I think I've mentioned that being tired is the worst feeling ever for someone who experiences mania. I just want to be wide awake and happy all the time, which obviously is unrealistic, but that's how good mania feels. Mania is great until you have to deal with the aftermath, which may include drugs or alcohol, excessive spending, or hyper-sexuality, just to name a few symptoms.

March 1, 2019

If you have ever had a real or perceived near death experience or something very traumatic, then you might find yourself thinking, "Wow. I can't believe I survived that.". I get these feelings a lot stemming from my hospitalizations and panic attacks. My life has been in jeopardy more than I would like for a 37 year old. In July, I will have survived my first breakdown for 13 years. When you piece together my story, maybe you will find it as amazing as I do a) that I survived at all, and b) that I made something productive out of my life. Not all of those years were good and enjoyable, but overall, I'm glad I'm still here. I know that life isn't fair, but I don't feel like I got a raw deal or anything like that. I have had an amazing life to this point, and I am grateful (most of the time).

I am proud of the positive impact I have had on others, and I have had some really great times, whether it be taking road trips to concerts or family vacations or just hanging with friends and family on a regular, boring, Ohio night.

When I was a kid, I was good at sports, and I dreamed of being a professional athlete. So much so that I would practice my autograph on notebooks and paper so that it would look great when I was signing autographs. I never thought I would be autographing books. When a shipment of my books come in the mail, I get a lot of joy from signing them. It's not an arrogant thing. It's just that I feel like my signature is a piece of me that goes with the copy of the book, and therefore the reader, wherever it goes. I guess that's a romantic idea, but I like to believe that part of me is in every autographed copy. My secret dream is for me to become famous, so that all my readers can sell my autograph for money. I know that's silly, but I always wished it would happen.

March 2, 2019

I had a weird experience last night. I took my nightly medication, and then I had a bowel movement. Sometimes after going to the bathroom, I feel extreme relief and happiness, almost. Not last night. I had some coffee before I went to the bathroom, so I assume that's why I had so much anxiety after I was finished. I had taken my medication already, so I just tried to stay occupied for as long as I could. I was having mild body and chest pains mainly. Racing thoughts too. There was a single beer in the refrigerator, so I thought I would try to have a beer to calm down. It doesn't usually work, which is why I rarely drink anymore, but it did last night. Almost immediately, I calmed down and felt the numbness of the alcohol. It made me remember why I used to self-medicate, and I felt a little guilty actually, which is silly. The beer tasted like it did when I was 16 years old since I rarely drink. I am going to remember that a single beer helped me, but I just have to make sure that I don't get in the habit of drinking to feel better. It's really only a problem when I drink to excess. The last time I did that was in October for my birthday, and I considered that a special occasion. I haven't had any outbursts like that since October, so I am confident in my almost complete sobriety. I have no moral objection to alcohol or marijuana. I just know that those substances are not good for me and don't give me relief like they used to. If drinking and smoking weed made me feel good, I would probably still do it honestly.

March 3, 2019

I had a small victory over my anxiety yesterday. In order for me to drive a car, I usually have to take medication and then wait for it to work before I can get behind the wheel without panicking. I had to go to the store yesterday about two miles away and there was still 45 minutes until my medication was due to be taken. I decided to try and drive, even though I hadn't taken my medication and was not due for another 45 minutes. It was definitely more difficult than usual, but I did it. Once I visited with the clerk, who is a friend of mine, and bought my items, it was time to take my medication. I just took my medication in the parking lot and had a cigarette until it started to work a little bit. I drove home with no problems either. I always thought it was strange that I have trouble driving because I used to deliver pizzas and drive for a living. Countless hours behind the wheel, and I'm basically back to being a beginner again. It's very frustrating because I will want to leave the house sometimes, but my anxiety prevents me from being confident enough to drive, or I have to wait for my medication to work to drive even the shortest distances. I have had major panic attacks while driving, but nothing major for a while. The worst it gets now is chest pains and neck stiffness, sometimes accompanied by brain fog or mild dizziness. Any driving over 5-10 minutes is an extreme accomplishment for me, and I have only been able to do it a handful of times in the last several years.

March 4, 2019

It seems like I always have anxiety to some degree. Most of the time it's manageable. I still have overwhelming anxiety and panic attacks sometimes, even with medication. I came up with a term that

I call, "hanging myself out to dry", where I wake up way before I am supposed to take my medication, and I end up having extreme anxiety or a panic attack. Sometimes I lay in bed or sleep just to avoid the anxiety of being up and about. Then, when I get out of bed, I am so exhausted that I reach for coffee. If I drink all of my coffee and there's a lot of time before my scheduled medication time, I can have a panic attack. I have been fighting this cycle for years, and it's actually called, "the vicious cycle of anxiety", which I think I already mentioned. It's a constant battle between being aware and awake and calm at the same time. My former doctor reduced my Klonopin by 50% almost immediately upon meeting with me, and it took some adjusting. Overall, I am functioning at a higher level, but I still have major anxiety setbacks and panic attacks. Like I mentioned, some of it is in my control with the caffeine intake, but sometimes like in the middle of the night, I can't really do anything about it except to ride it out, so to speak, until my next medication time. A good day for me is when my anxiety is manageable, and my bipolar symptoms are minimal.

Even if I have what some may call a bad day, I try to find the good in the day. It really helps me to stay busy and productive with my advocacy work or selling copies of my book. I feel like even if I am uncomfortable because of my anxiety that maybe I at least helped some people that day.

March 6, 2019

Anxiety is so uncomfortable, and it can be physically painful. I am experiencing anxiety right now, and it's hard for me to type this. My chest hurts, I'm itchy all over, and just generally sore all over my body, especially in my neck and shoulders. Panic is totally different. My mind races. I can't sit still, although I still get fidgety when I'm just slightly anxious too. Sometimes, my arms and legs will get weak or have a pins and needles feeling. With both anxiety and panic, minutes feel like days until I can get the relief from my medication. I can't help but to watch the clock. I am very strict about when I take my medication. I don't abuse it, and it's hard for me to take it even a minute early because of my OCD. There is almost no better feeling than when calmness sets in after a bout with anxiety or panic. Sometimes I even get goosebumps because it feels so good. Anxiety and panic upset my stomach so much that I may even have a bowel movement, although that could also be attributed to the caffeine in the coffee. I think I am a little extra anxious today because I have an appointment and an errand to run that both involve driving. I just took my medicine, so I am anticipating being calm enough to accomplish these things. In order for me to be successful, I just have to wait until my medicine kicks in. It's not something that I enjoy doing, but it is what it is, I guess. I wish I could come and go as I please, but it's just not always possible with my anxiety. It just takes some planning.

March 8, 2019

I'm sure all of you know that Dr. Phil has a talk show. The other day, a woman was being interviewed after she escaped a serial killer. She said something that stuck with me. Just paraphrasing here, but she said something like, "After all I have been through, I will find joy". I think that's a great perspective. I feel the same way really. Finding joy is all within reason I guess. As long as I am not causing harm to myself or others, I feel like I have every right to find joy. Of course, my mind makes that difficult sometimes, but I can usually find something that makes depression less severe, and I feel like there's always something to be grateful for. I like to do some pretty boring things--- watch golf, sit on my porch while it's raining or snowing, read books--- but these activities bring me joy.

There's also another saying that says, "Comparison is the thief of joy". With social media and the mainstream media and even something as old as magazines or the newspaper, we can sometimes find ourselves comparing our lives to others. A lot of my friends have pretty exciting lives. Some have what other people might think are boring lives. If there were ever a competition between myself and some of my friends on who lives a more exciting life, I would lose. That's fine with me. I spent so long doing exciting things and living in the fast lane, that at my age, I really just want joy, love, peace, and quiet.

March 10, 2019

It's Sunday. I'm really starting to hate weekends. I can feel myself slipping into a low depressive episode. I was happy and manic for about a month, so I guess this is the punishment I get. I am so full of rage and frustration, but my body is too sore to move. I wanted to write this before I took my medication because these feelings, even the body soreness, usually go away. Actually, one of the tricks I tell myself to get through the pain is to remind myself that almost all the horrible feelings go away. I feel like I don't have any friends, and I always feel a pressure to go out on the weekends, but I very rarely do. I don't have much in common with people my age. Most of the people I know are married with children, or they just drink alcohol all weekend.

It seems like technology is getting out of control too. I feel like so many people sit home and watch TV in the form of some sort of streaming service or however, but I can't just sit still for hours and watch. Most TV shows bore me. I enjoy sports, but even those get boring after so many days in a row. When people my age actually leave the house, they are on their phones using social media applications or taking pictures or videos.

Cell phones were just beginning to be popular when I was in high school. They were very rudimentary. Nothing like they are now. We had fun back then. We were more in the moment. We would hop in a car with no destination and just live for a day or two. No phones or cameras. Just frisbees and music mainly. I feel like those were the best days of my life, and nothing as fun is ever going to happen to me again. It's very depressing. It's hell getting old.

It's also hard to have a lot in common with people who don't deal with mental illness. It's not their fault, but they just have no clue. It consumes my life because it is my life.

March 12, 2019

In Ohio, twice a year, the time changes. We either "spring forward" an hour, or "fall behind" an hour. In the spring, the time changes by one hour moving forward, and that just happened. I have more trouble adjusting when we move the clocks backwards than forwards. I had a strange night of sleep last night. I don't know if I ate too much dinner or what. I was laying in bed watching TV, and I could feel my heartbeat in my neck. Every commercial made me anxious. It was a long, drawn out anxiety attack, rather than the sudden, potent panic attacks that I get. I usually sleep in clothes, so I took some off to get some cool air on my body. That seemed to calm me down, and I fell asleep. I had a nightmare that I was working one of my old jobs and I couldn't find where I had parked my car. When I have nightmares, sometimes they are more frustrating and exhausting than terrifying. I woke up in a cold sweat. I got up out of bed to have a cigarette and calm my mind, and that seemed to work the rest of the night. I feel much better now. It's about 3am, and I wanted to write this all down while it was still fresh in my mind.

March 12, 2019

I just want everyone to know that I don't have my shit together. I'm always smiling in my pictures, but sometimes I don't really feel like it. I joke around all the time because I like making other people smile and laugh, and it helps me deal with my life. Almost every day of my life I am struggling. The reason I mention this is because it's important to know that you aren't the only one who has bad days, or struggles, or you're not perfect. For the people who use social media, we can get caught up in comparisons, and a lot of people put on a face to make it seem like their lives are perfect. I just want you all to know that my life and personality is far from perfect. I try my best with what I have, and I am usually positive, but I just want you to know that you are not alone if your life isn't perfect.

Knowing that you are not alone is something absolutely critical with mental illness. Most of us are struggling, mental illness or not, and sometimes we are all guilty of only talking about all the good stuff on social media. On the other hand, I don't think it's cool to be sad, negative, vague, and nasty all the time on social media either. I think that social media is more powerful to our psyches than a lot of us know or would like to admit.

I don't know if this is a symptom of OCD, bipolar, or anxiety, but whenever I type something out, whether it be on social media or a text message, my brain repeats it several times. It becomes disturbing when the repetition just keeps going and going. I always thought that I had a photographic memory. When I took a test in school, it's almost like I could see the pages of the textbooks in my mind and just spit out the information. I was one of those people that usually understood the course material the first time through. In this case, it helped me. When it doesn't help me is when I wake up from a nap, and the same song lyrics are repeated over and over, sometimes for weeks. I have to immediately try to think of a different song because it's so annoying and disturbing.

It's very rare when there isn't some kind of "noise" going on in my mind. It's either song lyrics or something I just read or tasks that I have to do for the day. Caffeine just accelerates these thoughts until everything becomes jumbled and nonsensical. I don't know how else to describe these rapid thoughts as they make me feel like I am going crazy. More clinically, it is probably a form of psychosis, although "feelings of going crazy" is listed as a symptom of anxiety and panic. I try to focus on a single task or use a grounding technique to quiet my mind. It's amazing when my mind is quiet and I can truly relax.

March 16, 2019

I would rather not take medication, but I just have to. It's a part of my life now after almost 13 years. A lot of people have a negative view of pharmaceuticals, but I know that I am more stable when I take mine. I have only missed one dose in the last 13 years, and it was a total accident. One problem with bipolar people is that they start taking medication, and they feel better, so they stop taking the medication. This usually results in a full blown manic or depressive episode. I have been advised since the beginning to continue taking my medicine even if I feel good. Even when the medication made me feel awful, I trusted the process. Current day, sometimes my mind and body feel like they are on fire when it's time to take my medication. My medication helps me to calm my mind and body. They don't make me feel high, and it's not some kind of fun thing for me. At best, my medication makes me feel stable and able to deal with daily life. I also realized that I was at such a heavy weight that I needed to lose weight. In the last year, I have gone from 618 pounds to 565 pounds. I plan on continuing to lose weight.

Staying sober also helps the mind-body relationship. I have a terrible addiction to caffeine, but I've learned to work around it. I am a heavy cigarette smoker too. I roll my own cigarettes, which are supposed to be not as toxic as manufactured cigarettes. It's definitely cheaper. A pack of my cigarettes only costs 80 cents to roll myself versus about $7 a pack in the store. I'm also not stupid enough to believe in a safe cigarette, but it's really just damage control.

March 17, 2019

It's St. Patrick's Day. The coffee tastes extra good this morning, and I got some good sleep. Probably because I took a shower yesterday. It had been at least a week since my last shower. My grandfather, my mom's dad, who I never met, was buried on St. Patrick's Day, so today might be a little emotional for my mom. I had a length of time, and I don't remember how long the span was, but it seemed like I was calling for an ambulance frequently for panic attacks. I remember one time, the paramedics and cops showed up and I was hysterical. The TV was giving me messages that I thought were from God, and I hid a knife in the flower box outside because I thought there were people coming to get me. I think I was having paranoia and psychosis symptoms along with a panic attack all rolled into one bout.

Another time, my mom and I went to an outdoor music concert about 3 miles from my house. I drank a large margarita, and something snapped. I wanted to get on stage and announce that I was running for President. Luckily, my mom stopped me, but I was very angry at her. She threw a water bottle, and it almost hit me, and I became enraged. I told her to call my dad because I didn't want to ride home with her. My poor mom.

March 18, 2019

The promise of coffee usually gets me out of bed in the morning when I'm depressed. I don't suffer from depression too often because that's not the brand of bipolar disorder that I have. I am more likely to get out of bed from irritation, uneasiness, and the inability to lay still. Some of the most peaceful moments of my life are in my bed. It's awesome when I can just lay in bed with the lights off and think about nothing. This is a rare occurrence. Even if I only have a slight discomfort, it's relaxing. All four walls of my room are decorated with mostly sports memorabilia with some autographs from poker professionals mixed in. I love just laying in bed and looking at the walls. Any time my mind is quiet is a great thing.

This book has given me direction that I was looking for. Before this book, every day was starting to feel the same and I didn't feel like I was doing enough to stop the stigma surrounding mental illness, despite my social media page with almost 700 members from about 15 countries. I just want to be productive. I want to prove everyone wrong, even though I think most people would call my life a success story. I'm my own biggest critic, so maybe that's all it is. I think it's good to be productive and motivated and try to do something bigger than myself. I feel like if I write an entry in this book or work on my social media page, that can be enough for me for the day. I tell myself, "Well, at least I did something productive today even though I didn't feel well". My hope with this book, just like my other two books, is that people will find comfort and be inspired and find otherwise positive feelings from my writing.

Right now, my purpose is to be an advocate and to share my story. Maybe some day that will change, but for now, I am doing well in helping others catch a glimpse of what it's like to live with mental illness. I also hope that all my writing and advocacy has helped people with mental illness not feel alone.

March 19, 2019

When I was in high school, we were given an assignment to try and find out what our careers might be and what major to take in college. I really had no idea how to answer. I answered the most honestly that I could. I said I didn't care as long as I was happy. It seems to me that you either decide to go for money or be of service to others. Service jobs, like being a teacher, just don't pay as well as being a stock trader, for example. There are jobs that combine money and service like being a doctor, but in general, I think money and service are separate. Don't get me wrong. I enjoy material things to an extent, but I'm really very simple and frugal. The idea of trying to make money and acquire material possessions my whole life seems boring and empty to me. I need meaning and purpose.

When I chose psychology as a major in college, my plans were to go on to get a doctorate and charge people hundreds of dollars an hour and tell them how to fix their lives. Two years out of undergrad school, I went to the hospital and I was diagnosed with mental illness. I didn't know that I wanted a life of service until I was sick and then recovering.

Service is more important to me than money, but the world runs on money, so of course I still try to make money too. There has to be some kind of marriage or compromise for me. I dream of the day when I have a lot of money, not to spend, but to share. I don't find joy in expensive things, and I think they are wasteful. It doesn't matter to me if I live in a house or an apartment. It doesn't matter to me what kind of car I have, just so long as it runs. I don't need fancy clothes or food either. I think part of the reason I fell sick is because I was so obsessed with making money. Money is stressful. If I have to sacrifice money for peace of mind and my mental health, then so be it.

March 21, 2019

I had somewhat of a victory today. I had to run an errand about 5 miles from my house. I just had to drop something off. Normally before I drive, I have to take medication. Today I decided to challenge myself and leave to run this errand without taking my medication first. I took it with me in my pocket just in case I needed it. I take medication at certain times, and it was going to be time while I was out. I drove the short distance and ran the errand without taking my medication first. I was slightly anxious, but nothing that I couldn't manage. Later in the day, I had some pretty bad anxiety. I feel like I hold a lot of tension in my neck, and it's very uncomfortable.

    Whoever says that anxiety is just a feeling doesn't get it. It can be physically painful from stomach cramps, chest pains, to migraines to joint pain. That has been my experience anyway. Sometimes my anxiety is so overwhelmingly painful that I have to lay down in bed and allow my medicine to do it's thing. I remember what life was like without anxiety. I haven't been anxious my whole life. I think I started to get mild anxiety in high school and college, and it turned into major anxiety and panic attacks around 2008-2010, when I was about 28 years old. I'm trying to remember as much as I can, but understand that a lot of my memories are foggy and jumbled.

March 23, 2019

    Not everyone who says they are your friends are rooting for you. I know this sounds negative, but some people who say they are your friends would rather be more successful than you than see you win at life. Same thing goes with telling people your plans. If your plans don't fit into others' "boxes", they will find some reason why your plan won't work. Everyone has these theoretical boxes. The psychological term is basically called a schema. A schema is just the bare minimum of how we classify things in our brain. Think of flash cards. When you were young, you might have seen a flash card of a chair. This chair is your schema on what a chair is and what a chair should look like. Now, there a million different types of chairs. Based on your schema, you have to decide every time you see something that looks like a chair if it is a chair or not. When I say that people have mental schemas, if you will, it's not that hard to believe. If an opinion or idea doesn't fit someone's schema on how life should be, they won't believe in your plan or opinion.

 Cognitive dissonance is the uncomfortable feeling when facts challenge our schemas. Some people will believe in falsehoods just to protect their "boxes"/schemas. It's very hard to change a belief once you have believed it for so long. Most of you probably run into this every day, and it can be very dangerous to protect our schemas, even in the face of contrary facts.

March 25, 2019

 When I first got out of the hospital in 2006, I didn't really know what was going on for quite some time. Maybe even a few years. All I could do was eat and go to the bathroom. If I took a shower, it was like a miracle. When I started to become more coherent, little by little, I had a chip on my shoulder. I felt like I needed to prove myself to everyone that I was still capable of working and living a normal life. That this wasn't something I was faking to get out of having to work. I had a job since I was 15 years old all the way until the time I became sick, and I just thought that's how life was. You worked when you could as long as you could. I guess that's how normal lives go. I tried returning to work several times after I became sick, and the result was always some kind of mental breakdown, even to the point of hospitalization. I really didn't understand my illness very well or its limitations. Eventually, I would be approved for disability, and the feelings of having a chip on my shoulder returned somewhat. Most people who don't understand mental illness or disabilities in general don't have a high opinion of people who receive assistance from the government. After writing two books, and now a third, and having my advocacy work, I don't think I have much to prove to anyone anymore. Maybe the need for approval was all in my head to begin with. People who love me tried to understand, and why should I care what anyone else thinks? I think it's just human nature. I am also super competitive with high standards, which usually served me well, but maybe you could see how it could influence my self-image in a negative way. I was used to performing at a high level for basically my whole life, and then in a matter of days, everything came to a screeching halt. I am my own biggest critic.

March 26, 2019

Survive and advance. There's a large tournament going on right now to determine the National Championship of college basketball. It starts with 68 teams, and teams play each other in elimination games until there's a champion. Survive and advance is the unofficial motto of this tournament. That's how mental illness is sometimes too. Just surviving and getting to the next day or next resting period can be an accomplishment. Bipolar disorder is extremely unpredictable, but I have learned a few tricks and signs of when I need to rest or sleep. Anxiety and panic are somewhat unpredictable too, but again, I've learned a few things about what helps calm me down and what doesn't. Survive and advance. When I am going through some difficulty from my disorders, I try to have faith in my medicine and tell myself that eventually the pain will go away. I have to hang on for dear life sometimes, but I have done well over the last 13 years I guess. I don't know how to teach that. You have to be an extremely strong person. I wish I could bottle it up and give it away. I think a lot of it comes from how I was raised, but also just having that will to survive. It's an intangible. Not everyone has it.

I will never pretend to be a perfect person because I have my vices too. I'm lucky that they don't involve self-medicating with drugs and alcohol anymore. I'm definitely addicted to coffee and cigarettes, and I probably gamble too much. Food used to comfort me too, but I have broken that habit, and I have lost anywhere from 50-60 pounds. I don't know the exact amount because I don't keep track very well. I didn't want my whole life to revolve around food and my diet. I know I have to keep losing weight, but there's more to life than worrying if I eat some fast food or drink a soda or whatever the unhealthy food might be.

Today was a good day because I got out of the house to mail some things that I sold using the computer. There's a post office very close to my house, and my mom drove me there. The victorious part is that I didn't wait until it was time to take my medication. I accomplished everything and then took my medicine before the ride home. I can always tell when it's time to take my medicine because I am extremely irritable with little to no patience. I hate that I get that way because that's not who I am, but I figure if I can control it so that I don't bark at anyone that I have beaten it long enough for my medicine to work. Sometimes, my mania and anxiety make me want to jump out of my skin or go running down the street because it's so uncomfortable. It's like my mind and body can't contain that negative energy. I suppose this mega energy has served me well in the past when I was working a lot of hours and attending college at the same time. It's a fine line though before it turns into destructive mania. I try to be aware of my mood at all times, and I do an evaluation at the end of every day. How were my symptoms? Did I try my best? Was I productive? Did I handle stress well? I always try to find something positive to build on at the end of every day before I fall asleep.

March 27, 2019

One of the times I was hospitalized around 2010 was for mania and psychosis. I was admitted for the second time in my life. I remember a refrigerator full of cheese and apple juice that was comforting despite the atmosphere. I was only in there for 3 days, but I would join a Bible study group every morning just to read and reflect on life. It was very comforting. The leader said, "Just stick to Psalms and Proverbs", and I did. I learned a lot about wisdom.

We also played board games and made crafts. I still have some of the tinted glass that I made out of plastic cut outs and paint. My whole life has been Catholic education, and all I know now is that I am a servant to a higher power. It doesn't make a difference to me if it's a man, woman, or other being or just some kind of magic energy that is bigger, stronger, and wiser than I am. I don't need to put a title or name to it. Some people do, and that's fine, but a lot of harm has been done throughout history in the name of organized religion. I still believe in miracles, and a lot of people, including myself, would see my life as a miracle. I'm telling you, I've been so close to death so many times, that it can only be described as a miracle that I am still here, and I am grateful. It's not very cool or hip to be religious or spiritual, but I still pray anyway. Praying and living a life of servitude is a noble living even if there isn't anything bigger than us. I'm just trying to do my part. I've learned that what you reap is what you sow, and I guess that's a religious idea, but I am truly blessed in my life. I will admit that I forget sometimes. I get in bad moods. But it seems like that blessed feeling never really goes away.

March 30, 2019

Does it get better or do we just get used to it? I can't remember where I saw this probing question, but my answer is both. In the last few years, my symptoms have become more manageable, and generally, less severe. On the other hand, I have symptoms that occur frequently that I have just gotten used to. Body soreness, sweating, itching, chest pains, trouble driving, fatigue, depression, are some just to name a few. I think sometimes people have this expectation that they should feel perfect all the time with no troubles or pain. I accept that I have a mental illness and I may not feel well every second of every day. How I measure a good day is only partially based on my symptoms. I am more concerned if I am being positive, kind, humble, hopeful, and productive. Even if I am symptomatic throughout the day, I can still say that I had a good day if the previous mood and direction are met. I am not anti-doctor or anti-medication of course. My life relies on me taking medication and seeing a doctor. I just don't think it's reasonable to have an expectation of perfection when it comes to our health, even more so if you have a mental illness or some other type of chronic illness. There's going to be pain and bad days. I think it's just what level you can tolerate all the nagging bumps and bruises that being a human being entails. I have found that I am pretty tough, and I have a pretty high pain tolerance, but I'm not someone who can always bear the pain of mental illness. I need to take medication and naps to help recover. I need coffee to keep me awake and productive. I smoke cigarettes to manage my anxiety. I drink beer from time to time. I will say it again. I'm not a perfect person or a perfect picture of someone who deals with mental illness, but I try to give my best effort at all times.

April 1, 2019

I always like the feeling of a new month. It's like a clean slate. When I used to have to go to the doctor every month, now is about the time I would start to worry about the appointment, depending on what day it was. It's Monday, and the unpredictable Ohio weather has decided to turn chilly again. The Cincinnati Reds baseball team have started playing, so I always look forward to watching the games. Spring is just around the corner, which is always nice. I don't have much planned today, except for maybe one of my old friends might stop by to pick up some of my books.

I went out two days ago on Saturday night to a few of my favorite bars. I live in a small town, so I always run into people that I know. I actually met some new people this time. They seemed very nice, and they were interested in my books and story in general. A few of them bought copies on the spot. One of the guys has an audio set up where I could record my books to audio for people who prefer that medium. I never even thought about it to be honest. The guy who offered to help me explained that he had a mundane job, and he has dyslexia and ADHD, which makes it hard for him to read a book in print. He also mentioned that the last thing he wants to do when he gets off work is sit down and read a book. His phone records how much time he spends listening to audio books, and it was well over 5 weeks worth! Maybe I am missing out on an audio market.

April 2, 2019

My friend in college told me about a Philosophy class where the professor assigned an essay, and the prompt was simply "Why?". This friend told me that her friend handed in an essay that simply read "why not?", and received an A on the paper. I'm not sure if that story's true, but in my 37 years of living, I've found that there are generally two types of people: the whys and the why nots. The whys find every reason not to do something---the weather or financial cost, while the why nots are spontaneous and tend to say 'yes' to a lot more activities. I think it's a spectrum, and people vary from day-to-day. There are some people who are somewhere in the middle, and sometimes we are all cautious or throw caution to the wind, depending on our mood and other factors.

April 3, 2019

Sometimes it's one step at a time. One foot in front of another. Sometimes the road seems long if you get caught up in where it ends. It takes 4 years to graduate college, or it takes 2 years to do a job apprenticeship. Keeping the end goal in mind is good, but it can be overwhelming. With mental illness, it seems like it's always a baby steps approach, which can be quite frustrating if you are like me and tend to be an overachiever. I had to learn that progress is a process. One breath at a time even. If you can't move forward on a certain day, look back at how much you have accomplished. Even if you just survived mental illness for any length of time, it's an accomplishment. I understand that. A lot of people do. There are always going to be people who don't understand and look down upon people with mental illness. It's up to them if they will ever be cured of their ignorance. My reactions are the only thing in my control, and even then, I struggle to maintain calmness and courtesy in the face of insulting ideas about mental illness. Maybe my writing will help change some minds. Maybe people who suffer from mental illness will be comforted in knowing that they are not alone. Maybe someone doesn't quit because of my story. Whenever I hear feedback that my story influenced others in a positive way, it makes all the hard advocacy work, worth it.

I knew I had to lose some weight when I could barely get out of bed one morning due to body soreness. I was almost paralyzed from the soreness, and I had a panic attack from the restricted movement. I didn't really know what to do. I also saw a picture of me that really hit me hard, where I looked so huge and bloated. I have lines on the skin of my feet from where they used to swell. My legs used to swell in the summer heat too. Not anymore. I have lost about 70 pounds at this point, but I don't keep track obsessively, and I try not to obsess about it just in general. I weigh myself about 6 times a year. I also get body soreness from anxiety and panic attacks, but I have noticed a pretty significant positive difference. My blood pressure has gone down, and my resting heart rate is slower, both of which make my doctor happy.

I am more confident in the way I look too. I've been big my whole life, so I'm not so delusional to think that I will ever be skinny. I just want to be physically healthier, which I believe will contribute to a more healthy mental state as well. I don't know what my heaviest weight was either. I have been counting down from 618 pounds, so I'm about 70-80 pounds less than that now, maybe even more. I haven't weighed myself for several weeks.

Several years ago, I lost 144 pounds, but I gained it all back and then some. I'm a little mad at myself for getting out of control again, but sometimes physical attributes, including weight and hygiene, take a back seat to mental health. When I was really struggling with my symptoms, it was almost impossible to keep up with daily physical hygiene, and it wasn't much of a concern either. I have made improvements in physical hygiene, but I would like to do better. Taking a shower used to be near impossible at my heaviest because of the physical nature of the task, and I would get dizzy from claustrophobia. Those symptoms have improved also. I drink gallons of water a day, and lots of coffee. A few beers or a soda here and there. I substituted 2 bananas as breakfast every morning, and I eat smaller portions for lunch and dinner. No sweets or snacks. That's about it. Nothing too regimented. There are plenty of days when I eat too much, but I know if I get back to the base line of my diet, I will be fine. I'm not going to beat myself up during the whole weight loss process. I have tried the best I can, and that's always all I can ask of myself.

<u>**April 7, 2019**</u>

I used to think that my mental illness was a divine punishment handed down by God because I wasn't such a good person. I know now that it's not true. So much good has come from my experiences, even though it has been quite painful at times. Brains lie, especially if you suffer from mental illness. I get negative thoughts all the time. My brain says to me, "You are worthless", or "Your work doesn't matter" or "no one cares about you". After dealing with these thoughts for many years, I have to know that my brain is lying, and that these thoughts are not reality. It's always great when I hear that I helped someone. Not only does it help combat these false, negative thoughts, but it gives me a sense of pride and confidence. There is overwhelming evidence that these negative thoughts are false, but I still have them. It's the illness talking. The fact that I still have these negative thoughts, despite contrary evidence, just shows the power of mental illness.

Mental illness can defy truth and reality. Maybe describing mental illness as the brain lying may help understand how someone could be depressed or anxious, despite concrete, contrary evidence. It may also be easier to believe that mental illness is a brain malfunction rather than some kind of faultiness in thought.

April 8, 2019

Academics make sense to me. Poetry makes sense to me. Sports make sense to me. I understand a lot of things, but sometimes I am left confused by mental illness. I have everything I need, and an easy life for a 37 year old, at least as far as responsibilities go, but right now I am feeling a despair that my body can barely hold. The feelings of hopelessness, despair, and sadness despite concrete evidence that I shouldn't feel this way. Maybe part of my journey is to understand this sadness when it doesn't make logical sense. With this knowledge, I can relate to others and help them when they are going through the same thing. I'm still not sure if I believe that everything happens for a reason, but it definitely feels that way a lot to me. I had plans to do something tonight, anything, just something to get me out of the house, but I was sad and anxious and physically sore. I feel better now, and I have compromised with myself that at least I wrote a journal entry.

April 8, 2019

You probably know a "control freak". It's kind of a mean term for these people really because I believe it's anxiety and OCD, just like I have. I think I am probably a control freak to some extent, but I have run into some really bad cases. The people who think that their schedule is the only schedule. They are rude and boss people around if their schedule is deterred in any way. They don't say please, thank you, or excuse me. Stuff like that. It would be interesting to see if there's a study with a correlation among all these things and people with severe OCD.

There are 5 types of OCD. My brand is called an obsessional. For me, it means that I obsess over numbers, song lyrics, or errands I have to run for the day. I get even more agitated if I haven't had my medicine. I try to remain calm and kind when I need to get things done, or when there's a lot on my mind, but I fall short sometimes by being irritable towards others. I try to explain the situation and apologize when necessary. It helps to know that I'm not a mean person, so any meanness that comes from anxiety is absolutely symptoms of my disorders. I don't always have time to explain my whole life story when I get agitated, so a simple "sorry about that" will have to do.

April 10, 2019

    I have bipolar disorder? What's that? A mental illness? There must be some mistake. I didn't do anything wrong. Maybe I just got a bad batch of marijuana or something. My brain was injured like from a car accident? How? I need medication? Probably for the rest of my life? I don't understand. I'm so mad that my family brought me to the hospital. I was doing fine. I need to get back to work. There are bills to pay. I have to stay here? For how long? You don't know? I didn't realize I had signed my rights away to be treated until I was no longer a harm to myself or others. I am describing my first hospital stay in 2006. I didn't know if I would ever be released. What a terrifying experience. The nurses weren't exactly mean or friendly. Just kind of business as usual. Like they worked in retail or something. The meals were awful, and my order was usually wrong. I always wondered if the workers messed up my order on purpose to see how I would react. Maybe I was imagining it all from paranoia. It was hard to tell right from wrong, up from down.

April 10, 2019

It's hard for me to understand why people don't talk about mental illness more. When I was first hospitalized, a lot of people knew about it, so maybe that helped me be more open. It was much easier on me to talk about it as much as possible, and it still is. It's easier for me to tell people that I can't hang out because of my anxiety than to make up false excuses. Or if I am experiencing other symptoms, I just try to be honest about it. When people say there is a stigma attached to mental illness, what they mean is that there's a label or perception of people with mental illness. That they are "crazy" (whatever that means), or there is just something generally wrong with them. Maybe some people are embarrassed, and see mental illness as a personal failure. I think that's a common internalization. I can understand that I guess because I don't think I was always so forthcoming with how I felt. It's hard for me to remember all the time during my recovery. I guess I just learned over the years that being open and honest helped me more than pretending everything was okay. I also learned that sharing my story helped others who maybe weren't so open. I've had countless conversations, which I consider confidential, from people who were ashamed of their illness. I've had a lot of support too from friends and family, and even strangers with all my talking and writing. So all of that is positively reinforcing too. I am going to go through this one way or the other, so I might as well help people along the way.

April 11, 2019

My heart is full today. I saw one of my high school buddies for the first time in about 20 years. We traded war stories a little bit, and it was nice to have a visitor. I got to meet one of my best friends' daughter for the first time. I held her, and it was amazing. I cried a little, but I pulled myself together.

You are not a tree. You are allowed to move, and become someone different as you get older. I would hope so actually. We all make mistakes, but we shouldn't have to pay for them for the rest of our lives. Forgive yourself. Be the positive change you want to see in the world. Be kind. Be courageous. Don't be afraid to be great. Spread love and joy. Laugh as much as possible.

April 13, 2019

I read an article that talked about bipolar disorder as having a loud brain. This is definitely true in my case. Most of these journal entries are written before I even start typing because I have thought about the entries long before I actually start writing it down. A loud brain may be "cluttered" with song lyrics, or a to-do list, or just random thoughts. Writing my thoughts down helps clear out some of the clutter and make room for silence, if you will. Many therapists recommend people with mental illness keep a journal. I guess I finally understand why. Whenever I sit down to write, I can feel the burden of a loud brain go away, at least for a little while. At this point in my life, I've had the same TV commercial jingle stuck in my mind for at least a month. It starts right when I wake up. It feels like I can't control it. I do everything I can to think of something else or a different song. Maybe that's why sleeping is so relaxing for me. I have nightmares sometimes resulting from PTSD, but usually when I sleep, it allows my mind to be quiet and reset and regroup. Sleeping and naps also helps my body regroup from the general soreness that I experience from anxiety and my weight.

April 16, 2019

I rarely experience full-blown depression, but I do experience full-blown mania. I'm not an expert enough to know if there's a difference between bipolar depression and clinical depression. For me, when I start to feel depressed, I try to practice gratitude and think of as many positive things as I can. I think of my mood as a light switch. I try to flip the switch with as much positivity as I can when I feel that my mood is down.

A few years ago, I had a day where I was so depressed that I simply could not get out of bed and face my symptoms or the day. I still took my medicine as prescribed, but I just laid there all day. I was totally overwhelmed and exhausted. I haven't had a day like that since, but at the time, I told my doctor about it because I wasn't used to being so depressed. We monitored my progress in the next few months and it didn't happen again, so we just chalked that day up to having a depressive episode from bipolar disorder. While I personally may not experience depression often, I assume that other bipolar people do, and also people with clinical depression. I guess I am lucky in this way; however, mania is not much better. Yes, my mood is better, but the symptoms are very unpleasant: I can't sit still, brain fog, disassociation, money budgeting problems, excessive drinking or smoking, sleep disturbances, and chest pains. Those are just the symptoms that I can remember off the top of my head. I don't want this book to be like a textbook. I would rather just share my personal experiences with the knowledge and experience I have. If I need to quote or internet search something for accuracy, I will. I want readers to understand what my mental illness looks like on a daily basis, and not necessarily what a textbook contains, such as listing symptoms. I don't think listing symptoms that are common to my disorders really grasps the severity of the total package of disorders. It's probably worth mentioning here that for someone to have a disorder, he/she only has to exhibit MOST of the symptoms of that disorder, so you can imagine the differences within every disorder. If there are 10 symptoms, one person might have 7 and another person 8, but also the symptoms are different too. Mathematically speaking, there's a lot of variance and combinations.

April 17, 2019

Sometimes, when we get knocked down or when things don't go our way, it can be a good thing. Of course, at the time, it doesn't feel that way. However, there's not too many better feelings than saying, "I survived that" or "I got knocked down, but I got up". It helps prepare you for the next inevitable disaster than comes with living a human life. It builds character and confidence in your abilities. Maybe it gives you a purpose. I believe deep in my heart that I should be dead. That I'm living on borrowed time. I've internalized these feelings into gratitude and a higher purpose for living. Not every day is great, but I often find myself thinking how amazing it is that I survived everything. And I'm so proud of myself for never giving up. So much good has come from my disasters that it's hard to dispute that these disasters happened for a reason. I will let people argue about that. I'm not smart enough to know why things happen.

April 21, 2019

It's Easter Sunday. My parents are at Mass, and they are going out to brunch later. I admire their faith. They rarely miss Sunday Mass. I'm not anti-God or anything. I just try to stay away from religion or thinking too hard about if there's a higher being greater than humans. I have thought that I heard the voice of God or perhaps angels, and it scared the hell out of me, so maybe you can understand why I stay away from it all. I also think that it's impossible to really know as a human on Earth. Many people think they know, and a lot of people think they are sure that there is no God. I don't buy any of that, but I do believe that there are things beyond our understanding. Maybe humans are supposed to not understand some things. It's impossible to know everything, right?

I just don't understand why companies and governments spend money on obscure technology and space programs, when we have humans on Earth who are hungry, homeless, and diseased. There was a stand-up routine by a comedian named Chris Rock, who said, "There's no money in the cure. There's money in the medicine." I believe him to some extent.

April 22, 2019

"Do what makes you anxious". Some of the last advice my last doctor gave me before he moved on to his private practice. I thought HE was the one who needed help. At the time, I couldn't figure out how I was supposed to do anything when I had chest pains, sweating, fatigue, itching, and too nervous to drive. However, he was right. Things are getting easier for me. At least leaving the house and taking showers are. It's not a gold medal in the Olympics, but it's more progress than I've had in a while. I have left the house 3 times in the last week, and I have taken a few showers. I am up late at night, so I usually visit with friends at the bar or local pubs. I have to watch myself, and I am always fully aware of the problems I've had with drinking alcohol in the past. I can have a few with little problems, but that can easily turn into a lot and more frequently.

When I started going out more and being more social, I took a bit of a leap of faith. It's not that I really felt better. It's just that staying home anxious all the time was more painful than taking a chance on more freedom. I'm a bit of a gambler, but my mental health is something I usually don't gamble on. How much am I willing to risk in the name of recovery and wellness? The answer is a lot because really, what do I have to lose? My bed will always be there if I need to rest. I got tired of watching life go by through a foggy glass window. I was willing to risk the comfort of stability for a chance at more freedom. So far, it's working out.

April 23, 2019

After I take my medicine, no matter which medicine or time of day, if I don't feel some relief in an hour or so, I have a panicky moment where I question if I took the right combination of medicine and dosage. I don't think I've ever made a mistake of that nature, but it's just something I've done for as long as I've been taking medicine. I don't expect to feel perfect necessarily after my medicine, but I do expect some relief. If I don't feel that relief, I panic a little, but not a full blown panic attack or anything. Sometimes, I am just simply tired. My symptoms seem to be enhanced when I'm tired, and I know it's time for me to take a rest or even fall asleep for a few hours. My mind and body only work well in spurts of time. It's been this way for a very long time. Most of the time, I know what I can handle, and when it's time to rest. If I do too much, I get symptomatic and manic. I try to stop that cycle as soon as I can. The tricky part is being honest with myself and identifying mania, instead of riding the euphoria and continuing to be ultra-productive. I have to put a stop to my mania whenever I can because a manic episode can lead to self-medicating and otherwise destructive behaviors.

April 24, 2019

Technically, my relentless sense of humor is a defense mechanism, which has a negative connotation to it. I was joking around just days after I thought my brain had exploded in 2006. It helps me deal. It's one of the last bits of dignity that I have left. Being negative is one of the easiest things to do. I understand depression. I have lived with it. I understand that sometimes there's not much you can do to have a positive outlook. When you are depressed, it's very annoying to get unsolicited advice on how to "snap out of it". Take a walk. Go exercise. Write in a journal. Whatever cure these people think they have. A lot of times, they mean well, it's just that they don't understand severe depression. They probably have never experienced it. They confuse being sad sometimes with a brain malfunction that will not allow positive thoughts or energy to do any of these cures. But for every day life, depression being an exception, I had to practice being positive. My way of being positive is to joke around, even at my own expense. I am confident enough to make fun of myself.

When I don't feel like smiling or laughing, I feel like if I can give that joy to others, then my time is not wasted. If I can't laugh myself, let others laugh and be joyous. It can be infectious too. If I can make others laugh and smile, that rubs off on me. It's a gift that gives back. I have always been somewhat rebellious, so joking and laughing in the face of adversity feels like I am giving the metaphorical middle finger to my troubles. Dealing with my life in this matter may be my greatest personality trait.

April 25, 2019

I'm all caught up in my feelings for some reason. Usually happens after calming down from anxiety....there was a time when the medication wouldn't allow me to feel anything. Maybe pain at the most. I barely had any thoughts. Numb and thoughtless. I can't remember how long I was like that, but even bullshit symptoms feel good in a way now. Anything but numb and indifferent. I pulled myself out of that somehow and decided I was going to fight. So I ask you, are you going to fight or are you going to quit?

April 28, 2019

Life was passing me by, and it was killing my spirit. I would just watch everyone else living life with no issues, and it was depressing. It felt like my anxiety and panic would never get better. It's getting better, and I can only guess why, but I'm extremely grateful. I've tried to practice gratitude and positivity through everything. I think that has really helped me. I deserve credit for losing weight, and only missing one dose of medicine in the last 13 years. I took my medicine even when it made me feel awful. I trusted in the recovery process when I didn't have faith in it or the doctors. I will never be cured of my illness, but I don't have to be a slave to it. Some people probably think I'm crazy because I'm enthusiastic sometimes for seemingly no reason. I have a reason.

Life is the reason. I'm so thankful to even be able to drive myself to the store and buy a soda. Or go to a bar and hang out with friends. I was a prisoner to my anxiety for so long that every little fun activity I can do is probably ten times more fun for me than someone who doesn't suffer from anxiety.

I've been like a football coach to myself for so long in that I have to give myself pep talks and keep myself motivated, even when life is getting the best of me. I get excited to drink coffee on my porch. I get excited to run errands in my car. I used to have trouble even making eye contact with other people. My chest hurt, and I would get dizzy in open spaces or enclosed spaces, like the shower. I have to take a little credit for losing weight, being medicine compliant, and just generally not giving up.

I share my struggles and my story because I want to give others hope that it can get better. I have also been humbled through this whole recovery process. I don't take the good times for granted. If I am feeling well, I try to take advantage and do something fun or get out of the house. That way, when I am not feeling well, I have the good times to keep in mind while I am struggling. It gives me hope and faith that things will get better. In the back of my mind, I think that all my progress can be gone tomorrow, so I have a bit of a "carpe diem" (seize the day) personality. There has to be some kind of balance between planning for the future and living for today, but when you have a mental illness, long-term planning is difficult. It's hard to see the future because mental illness is a constant, relentless, daily battle.

April 30, 2019

One of the best compliments I have ever received was from my own mother. She told me that I was stronger than her. My mom has survived cancer twice, raised 5 children, lost over 120 pounds after age 60, and has generally worked her butt off for half a century. My mom is one of my heroes.

May 1, 2019

I don't have pleasant dreams. I don't know if nightmare is the right word exactly. When I dream or have a nightmare, it's always about school or work. I was embarrassed to go to school all the way through college because the desks were not big enough for my large body. I felt trapped and bored. I used to work a lot and go to college full time at the same time, so I was always on the go. A lot of the time I was manic at the least, and psychotic at the worst. So I have these nightmares where I am constantly working and on the go. I wake up relieved, but exhausted. It feels like my mind has been running for hours when it should be shut down and resting. I guess a loud brain can translate into the unconscious too. I don't really have nightmares about the hospital too much, but I have flashbacks while I am awake, which are even more terrifying. Triggers such as the doctor's office or anything medical on the news or a TV show really make me squirm.

May 5, 2019

I've had several weird dreams/nightmares over the last few days. It seems like I am always at work or school. Then, there's the flat out weird category. So the first dream I remember is I am working at the pizza place where I had my first psychotic break in 2006. A guy gets his tongue stuck in the pizza over conveyor belt, and the owner has to cut his tongue to get him out. For some reason, I don't remember being grossed out or panicking. I think I dream about work because I have had several breakdowns from working long hours at jobs. Kind of a PTSD-type thing.

The other dream is just weird. I was a Batman-like character where I could climb walls. I was trying to get away from some kind of enemy. That was really the whole dream, but it seemed to drag on and on. Most of my dreams are similar in that they are exhausting. Very repetitive. I wake up, and I am so relieved the dreams are over because I feel like I had just run a marathon. My dreams aren't really scary, but rather just weird and confusing.

May 8, 2019
NEW POEM
5-8-2019

I've been gone for so long
I don't know my way back.
My dreams are golden,
But all I see is black.
It's hard to tell what is real and what is not.
My memory is distorted and surreal.
I just live by what I see and feel.
I tried to join the race,
But my legs were in glue.
I've done the best that I can do.

I think I have one more run left in me,

Before I finally give in.

Although that's how I felt last time

And the time before that.

I feel like I am living on borrowed time,

And that I have cheated death.

I guess we never really know.

Everything will pass in the end.

Family and friends.

It's all part of the ride I surmise.

A happy ending would be a nice surprise.

May 10, 2019

Money is always a hot topic when it comes to happiness. It seems like everyone thinks that money equals happiness or that it automatically brings happiness. I've heard sayings like, "It's hard to be sad on a jet ski", and things of that nature. I've had more money than I could spend before, and yes, I was happy because it bought me things that made me happy. I just can't help but think that I'm 37 years old, living with my parents, and I have $11 to my name. I'm still happy. I don't know if it's a mindset, or the fact that I feel like my life has purpose and value, not just to me, but to all the people I help with my books and mental health advocacy. Maybe purpose equals happiness. Maybe gratitude equals happiness. Maybe it's all of these things, including money. All I ever wanted in a career was to be happy. I really didn't care if I was a garbage man or a professor. I just never understood what there was to life except happiness. I certainly don't have all the answers, but the fact that I can be happy with lots of money or a little money suggests that it's not money that makes me happy. I think money helps you to be happy to the extent of not being stressed out over bills. Financial security or stability with your necessities could equal happiness. I'm extremely grateful that I have that. I will probably never go homeless or hungry, but I'm also humble enough to know, that "the poor house is right around the corner", like Regis Philbin's mom used to tell him. This is stuff I think about. "The unexamined life is not worth living" after all. Money isn't going to take my symptoms away. If I had a lot of money, I'm not going to be able to magically drive my car without anxiety. Maybe I can be happy with little because I don't have a choice right now.

May 11, 2019

There are many stigma associated with mental illness. Stigma is basically a form of discrimination, prejudice, or labeling of someone with mental illness. Pill shaming is one such stigma. This is when someone is meant to feel inferior or guilty for having to take medication to help manage mental illness. This rarely happens with physical conditions. For example, many people accept that people with heart conditions need heart medication to survive, but there may be a stigma when someone with a mental disorder needs medication to survive and function. I'm lucky that I have never run into this, but people may say things like, "Have you taken your medication today?" when an argument arises, which is basically a cop out to minimize that person's feelings and make them invalid.

There is another group of people who think that holistic or natural remedies are sufficient enough to control mental illness. They may think that exercise and vitamins are enough. Personally, I take 3 different medications a day, which adds up to about 10 actual pills a day. I don't know anyone with a mental illness that doesn't take medication to some degree. I know people that take over 40 pills a day, which I think is a lot, but I'm not a doctor either. As a general rule, being supportive and minding your own business are good rules to live by when it comes to how someone is medicated. If the concern is coming from a loving place, that person will be more inclined to listen to your opinion about how he/she is medicated.

May 12, 2019

It's Sunday, and it's Mother's Day. I could go on forever about how much I love my mom and how much she has helped me, but I want to write about an anxiety obstacle that I overcame today. I went out to eat at a restaurant. It was always so difficult for me for a lot of reasons. I would be anxious on the car ride to the restaurant. I was physically exhausted, so sitting for an hour for a meal was overwhelming. I have anticipatory anxiety, which means that when I anticipate something is going to happen---like when the waitress brings out food---I get anxiety. It's not that I'm spoiled or especially hungry. The waiting was causing me anxiety. My paranoia would tell me that everyone was watching me eat. It's not true. I'm a messy eater too, but most people don't care what you are doing as long as you aren't causing a scene. A room full of crowded people would make me anxious and disoriented. Not today. For whatever reason, I was able to overcome all of these usual symptoms and actually enjoy myself. It could be that the timing was just right with my medication, or maybe I was able to muster up the strength because I wanted to do something nice for my mom on Mother's Day. Every time I conquer situations like this, I gain confidence. When I am confident, I am more likely to step outside my comfort zone and try more things that used to make me anxious in the past. It's a self-feeding process, where feeling "normal" and enjoying myself are the rewards. Maybe I wanted to show my family that I am getting better too. Maybe I needed that feeling of accomplishment. It's good to test the waters of anxiety every so often because if I succeed, it just adds more confidence, and it's a very positive step in my recovery.

May 13, 2019

Social media posts:

For me, it hurt worse to stay the same than to try and make a change. I was tired of feeling trapped in my own home with anxiety, panic, and depression. It took a lot of therapy, medication, a leap of faith, and brass balls, but I'm finally starting to taste freedom again. Thanks to everyone who supports me, in every capacity. Much love from the bottom of my heart.

So I'm thinking about making the drive downtown to JACK Casino in Cincinnati. I only have $15, but it's really more of a driving exercise/anxiety obstacle test. Anyway, some of you have heard my crazy gambling stories, so here's one I can tell on social media....

The first time I ever went to a horse track, I went with a few knowledgeable buddies. You get a program with all the races, horses, and other statistics when you get there. I guess as a way to feel like you are making educated guesses. I think it was the second horse bet I had ever placed in my life. I bet $2 on a straight trifecta, which is guessing the correct order of the first three horses, in exact order. For example, a straight trifecta 1-2-3, is 1 coming in first place, 2 coming in second, and 3 coming in third, in that exact order. They are very rare and lucky. Well, my ticket was something like 5-11-6, and it came in. My buddy says, "That might be a good one". I'm thinking $20 at the most or something. I have no idea really about any of this. I took the ticket up to the cashier, and it paid out $1,111 LOL. We had fun at the bar that night. Money was definitely flying around.

May 16, 2019

When I chose psychology as a major in college, my plan was to go the distance and get a doctorate. I thought I was going to solve everyone's problems and make a ton of money while doing it. Because everyone else had problems. Not me. When I couldn't continue school, I went to real estate school and earned my license. I passed the state test on the first try. I thought I was going to make a ton of money selling houses and such. That didn't work out either. Then I got sick and everything changed. I became a mental health advocate and eventually an author, twice. I was always a little bit of a poet, but I started sharing my work with people. I thought drinking and smoking weed would always be a part of my life. They're not. I'm almost always sober, and don't really enjoy either substance anymore.

My point is that almost nothing worked out as planned for me, but I'm satisfied with the mark I've made on the world. I rarely have money either, and I used to always chase the next dollar. I'm not like that anymore. I'm happy with the person I've become, and it's all because I failed and things didn't work out. I guess what I'm trying to say is keep working hard. You never know when things are falling into place when they feel like they're falling apart.

May 17, 2019

Today was a not-so-gentile reminder of why people with anxiety are true warriors. This is going to sound weird, but it is what it is. I have no science to back this up, but sometimes, after a bowel movement, my anxiety or mania kicks into action. I think it's because the toilet time is around when I take my medication. I purposely didn't take my medication any earlier because I really wanted to feel it so I could write about it, and explain it to people who might not understand. So, I used the toilet, and there was still about an hour until my medication time. I have made my medication times set in stone, but really it's supposed to be as needed. The bathroom complications and medication times are both a result of my OCD. Anxiety is different for everyone, but here is how my anxiety/panic bout went just now. The muscles in my neck tense up. My chest hurts. I started sweating, so I put on deodorant. My ears are plugged from the neck tension. I start having swallowing and breathing difficulties because I think I might pass out. Random thoughts and numbers are running through my head, and none of it makes sense. It's just noise. Is it bipolar or anxiety or both?

There is a symptom of bipolar called a "loud brain", where basically this is how the brain functions sometimes in a bipolar person. I have tingling in my arms. My stomach is in knots, and it's hard not to lay down. I start thinking if this is what death is going to feel like. I have flashbacks of the hospital and how awful those experiences were. I go outside for some fresh air, and everything is so fast and loud. It comforts me to see my dad gardening. Everything starts to slow down a little. I finally can't take anymore, and I take my medication 4 minutes early. It takes about an hour for it to fully work, but I can feel it within a half hour usually. My back is also tense. My face flushes. It's hard to sit still. It's hard to focus. I need to keep drinking ice water to quench my thirst and to keep me calm. I start rummaging through my baseball card collection to try and distract my mind, and I also start rolling cigarettes just to do something mindless and repetitive. One of my medication times is 10:30am. It is now 10:51am. I can feel the medicine working, the familiar sand in the eyes feeling, and I am starting to calm down.

This will give you an idea of what I have to do to maintain my stable mental health. I am not always stable, but stable so much as I do not have to be hospitalized. I have a lot of good things to report to the experts. I have been going out more, and driving more. I used to not be able to drive at all or leave the house. I also used to not be able to sit still at all or make eye contact with anyone. That's the kind of stuff that only shows up on the charts of my doctor.

A clinical diagnostician is going to stop by the house today to discuss a treatment plan for me for the next 3 months and beyond. Points may be something like testing my anxiety by driving, or go out and be social. Others may include better personal hygiene or helping with chores around the house. This is a fairly painless experience. I just have to manage my anxiety at the time of the appointment and during talking to the diagnostician. It really helps that he/she is coming to the house.

Today is Monday, and on Wednesday, I have my 3 month check up with a nurse practitioner. I have to go to a clinic close to downtown Cincinnati, and get refills on my medications and answer questions, which include, "Have you felt like hurting yourself or others?" or "Any drugs or alcohol?". When I have to travel this far from the house, it gives me extreme anxiety. It also gives me anxiety to be around so many people who are mentally sick. The whole process is physically and mentally exhausting. I used to need a few days to recover, but now I really only need a nap for a few hours to recenter myself. I have really thrived in the 3 months since my last visit. I used to have to see a doctor every month. It seems like I was always worried about the next appointment or recovering from the last appointment.

I also get checked by a clinical nurse, but all she/he does is check my blood pressure and weight. This nurse also asks general questions about my physical health. This nurse is always happy to hear about my weight loss and increased activity, and not so happy about me smoking. You have to pick your battles sometimes.

May 21, 2019

I always sign my books with my name and "Love and best wishes". I absolutely mean it with every part of my being. I don't hate anyone or wish ill will on a single person walking this planet. Not even people who have done me wrong. The people who have betrayed me are few and far between, and I will never forget who those people are. I'm not sure you can truly forgive someone unless you can forget, but the best I can do is just wish everyone well and good luck. I don't take it lightly when I tell people that I love them, or call them brothers. I don't really call my girl friends, sisters, but I tell a lot of people that I love them. It's not because I throw the words around in a meaningless way; it's because I mean it. I mean it as much as anything I have ever said. It's the highest level of friendship, love, and care that I have to offer. I give my heart away, and it has only backfired a few times. If being a loving person gets me hurt every once in a while, so be it. I'm not going to let a few bad apples ruin what I feel in my heart. So when I write these corny entries about wishing everyone love and success, I mean it. I feel it throughout my soul. So, in absolute seriousness, I wish you all good luck and much love!

May 22, 2019

I feel bad because the only time I talk about my dad on social media is to make fun of his mannerisms. My dad was hard on me as a kid. He still is, and I'm 37 years old. Maybe he knew that's what I needed. I'm extremely grateful that he was now. I will never forget, in grade school, I brought home straight As on my report card. He looked at it for about 10 seconds and said, "Well, there's always room for improvement". It hurt pretty bad at the time, but it's kind of funny now. That's just how he is. He wasn't the "hug it out" type dad. He was the authority of the house, and he expected respect. Rightfully so, because he worked every hour his job had to offer. Swing shift. Overtime. Whatever. He was always working to provide for us. He was in the National Guard Reserves during the Cuban Missile Crisis. I know he would have fought if he was called upon. Both he and his dad (my grandpa, WW2 vet) love this country, and would have definitely fought for her. Sometimes, I will tell my dad that I love him just to make him uncomfortable haha. I was upset one time that he didn't ever say those 3 magical words and he said something like, "You should just know". Okay. That settles that.

All of that bragging brings me to today. He is going to pay to have my truck fixed, and I can pay him back a little every month. He totally saved me on this one, and he has a track record of doing that. He has helped me so many times financially, especially through college. I have paid him back only a small amount of what he has spent on me. Another thing I want to add is that even though he worked so much, he still found time for my baseball games and practices, fishing, and golf with me. He didn't really care for the other sports that I played, so my mom was the parental support at those sporting events.

When I say that my dad and I are Cincinnati Reds fan, I can't tell you how much I mean that. We take it very seriously, and we know a lot about the game. It's how we have bonded since I was 5 years old. Just want to say how grateful I am for my dad for a change, instead of complaining about his mannerisms. The things he does that irritate me seem pretty small after everything he has done for me.

May 23, 2019

I've had 3 psychological evaluations in the last 3 days. It has been hard on my anxiety, but I managed it well. I had to see the doctor to have my medication refilled, and all of the appointments centered around goals for the future and a treatment plan for the next year.

My doctor does not like prescribing "benzos" like Klonopin, which I take, but it works for me. He knows I don't abuse it or take extra. At my appointment, he wanted to let me know that in the future, it could cause Dementia or Parkinson's Disease. I felt like saying, "Look buddy, I can't believe I'm still alive, so it's hard for me to worry or care about what might happen in 40 years". I've thought I was a goner so many times. I don't know if I've ever actually been close to dying, but that's how I perceive it, and that's what my attitude is. It's the best gift that mental illness has given me: Gratitude, humility, and appreciation for the "little things", like just waking up in the morning, or drinking coffee on my porch in calm and peace. I've learned to be more positive, despite bouts of depression (at least after I've had my coffee). I'm not a religious person, mainly because the thought of higher powers frightens me, but blessed is the best word I can think of to describe how my life has turned out. I may not be religious, but I realize that life is bigger than just mine.

After everything I've been through, the fact that I have had a positive impact on others in the slightest bit is amazing and hard to explain away with logic. I have bad days. I'm not saying that. But even in my bad days, I just think about the fact that I don't have to worry about food, clothing, or shelter. Probably never will. I'm already richer than 25% of the world's population. It's keeping my life in perspective like this that helps me through hard days. On top of that, I have so much support, and so many people rooting for me.

I've also learned the difference between wants and needs. I have everything I need. If I want anything beyond that or if I am lucky enough to have more than I need, I'm so appreciative. I just don't see life like a lot of people. Or maybe people just don't talk about it as much as I do.

May 28, 2019

I had some anxiety the other day, and I was laying in bed, watching TV, trying to calm down. There was a commercial that mentioned Spokane, Washington. I almost laughed because Washington is so far away from Ohio, and I'm struggling to run errands 2 miles away. It was a little depressing to think that I may not be able to travel far from home, but I also have awesome memories of road trips to music festivals and family vacations. I'm glad I traveled when I could.

May 30, 2019

I have a terrible habit of feeling like I have to finish leftover food. I've been fighting the urge through my weight loss pretty well. I also feel like I have to fill my coffee cup to the top and finish until the last drop. I didn't sleep well last night, and I noticed I was a little anxious. I filled my coffee cup to the top as usual, but I dumped out at least half so I can go back to sleep. This is a real struggle for me.

June 3, 2019

I don't like when mania is described as a high. I'm an old pot head, so when I think of high, I think of being stoned and enjoying myself. Mania can be enjoyable, but most of the time, it leads to destructive behaviors, such as sexual promiscuity, self-medicating, and poor money budgeting. The worst mania I ever had was in 2006, and it was accompanied with psychosis, so I was also delusional and having auditory hallucinations. It was just non-stop energy and racing thoughts, along with wild ideas about hearing messages.

These messages were directive, which means they were telling me to do something or go somewhere. Everyone has an inner dialogue, but directive, auditory hallucinations are completely different. Back in 2006, my thoughts were so jumbled and racing, and every so often, I would get a clear, directive message. Surprisingly, I remember how that felt, but it was like I was watching myself in a movie. I had no control over my actions.

June 6, 2019

This should be my last book. I am hoping that it will continue to educate people about mental illness, and maybe fill in some gaps in my story from my first two books. Mental illness is a daily struggle, and within every day, there are several small battles. It's almost impossible to escape. Most of my days are good and productive, and I have bad moments some days, but mental illness is always there. What I am getting at is that I'm getting a little burned out with all of it. I have to deal with mental illness every day, and then I am constantly writing and talking about it. My story even comes up a lot in casual conversation when I go out to have fun. I also run a social media page devoted to mental health, and I make at least 5-10 posts a day to try and help others. I'm hoping this book will bring everything full circle and maybe I can take a break from the advocacy work, even if it only for a short time. I want to focus on distributing my books. I just want there to be more to my life than mental illness and advocacy, even though it has been my passion for about 7 years. I'm looking forward to publishing this book, and then maybe taking a break from writing and social media, even if it is only for a week or two.

June 10, 2019

Overall, I am getting better if I compare my condition to the last couple years. It's truly an amazing story, but with progress, comes expectations. I worry that people are going to rely on me more, which is more pressure to function at a higher level. This is a pretty common feeling for someone who is recovering from mental illness actually. There are still days where I am too anxious to drive and completely sore from head-to-toe from anxiety and depression. There are days when I feel extremely blessed, and there are days when my attitude leaves something to be desired. Even my recovery has been bipolar, if you will.

Recovery can be a very slow, piecemeal process. It's extremely frustrating at times, but also very rewarding when I accomplish something new. A lot of things for me have taken a long time to achieve, and for me, there's nothing worse except for no progress at all. It seems like everything is a baby step process that I have to work towards. I just want everything to be better overnight. I have no idea how I have had the will power for almost 13 years now. Through having mental illness, I have found my calling and purpose. I have found the why. I still don't know or understand the how, and I try not to think about it too much. When I do think of everything I survived, I just say a little prayer of thanks to anyone who may be listening.

June 13, 2019

I posted this on social media, and I received a response from a friend of a friend:

Is there anything you want to know about mental illness or my condition specifically? I am looking for ideas for journal entries in my book. I have a small writer's block.

Friend's response:

- Here's an idea. I'm bi-polar like you. Have been on several different medications over the years. It's a real challenge to find the right one. How did you decide what was right for you? When to stop looking for something that worked better? Depakote worked great for me, but I was walking around in a haze, was like I was drugged. Took Abilify for a while. It kind of worked. I'm rapid cycling and it definitely took the "spikes" out of my mood swings, but was far from controlling them. Trying something new now, but to keep switching is tiring to say the least. How did you decide what was "good enough?"

My response:

I have to first say that I only have a Bachelor's degree in psychology with almost 13 years experience. Technically, I am not qualified to give counseling advice, but here is what I replied:

> That's a really tough question...I have been on the same combination of medications for about 8 years or so. I was having to go to the hospital for panic and paranoia quite frequently, and those visits stopped, so I guess I was pretty satisfied with that. There's no magic pill, and it's hard to say whether you will ever feel like you did before. You

might never feel "normal" again. It all depends on the person. Ultimately, it's your personal feelings about how much you think you can function, but also maintaining that stable balance. I think stability is the ultimate goal, and I think you will be happiest when that happens. I still have some pretty tough days, but I know overall, that I am a lot better than even a few months ago.

That's such a good question, and I think a lot of people think the same thing.

Everyone is different. Some people live with bipolar disorder and live somewhat normal lives. Some people can't get out of bed or leave the house.

Being stable is probably one of the most boring things for people like us. We just want to be "up" and happy all the time. I think the only way to effectively deal with this illness is to be stable most of the time.

June 17, 2019

It's Monday today. I told myself I was going to rest and not work, but that didn't work out so well. Some of my best productivity comes when I tell myself I'm not going to work. Maybe it's reverse psychology on myself. On Friday night, I went to a local bar for karaoke night. I had a great time and met up with some good friends. It's odd that getting up and singing in front of people doesn't bother me, considering so many other things irritate my anxiety. Maybe it's an energy dump/release for me. I've been singing karaoke since I was old enough to go to bars. Maybe I like the attention too.

I had a few beers, which is rare for me. I always have to make sure that I am not drinking to excess, and I didn't. When I go to a bar, I usually drink soda or water because alcohol is usually wasteful in combination with my medicine, and costly. My medicine is designed to keep me level, and alcohol is the antithesis of that, so they kind of cancel each other out. I have to drink a whole lot of alcohol to even get a buzz, and I'm usually not willing to do that. I made an exception at my birthday party in October, but like I said, I really have to watch myself. I never knew if I had a drinking problem, or if I was just self-medicating. I guess it doesn't matter.

As I was leaving, a guy who said he had just turned 30 years old, started a conversation with me. He said he was from Boston, and he was nice enough I guess, but I could tell he wasn't from the neighborhood.

My left eye is about half-closed, and I really don't know what happened. It burns too occasionally. This guy from Boston asked me if I had a stroke, and if I had ever considered losing weight. Pretty rude if you ask me. I guess he wasn't being mean about it, but it caught me off guard. Where I come from, you don't comment on someone's appearance unless it's a compliment. He did give me a high five when I told him that I had lost 60 pounds. People can be so rude. I don't come from a rich neighborhood, but most of us at least have manners.

Sunday was Father's Day, and my parents had my family over here for dinner. Family functions like this drain me, but I handled myself pretty well. I remember when crowds or a large number of people were extremely hard on my anxiety, so I guess I should be grateful that I can handle it now. I also told myself that I was going to enjoy solitude for the next few days, but I don't know if that will last. The last few weeks have been tough and busy for me.

June 19, 2019

Only a handful of my friends know how bad of a condition I was in almost 13 years ago, and for a few years after that. I've even made a lot of progress from just a few weeks ago. It seems like there's an ebb and flow to my condition. Makes sense, considering the dual nature of bipolar disorder.

I'm reading through my previous entries in this book trying to get it ready to be published, and I am almost moved to tears with gratitude. I look back at everything I have overcome, and it just hits me hard every so often. I'm so grateful to be alive, much less making a positive impact on other people. I know that this is how my life was supposed to turn out, and it's a great feeling. I don't wonder about my purpose anymore. Sharing my story is undoubtedly my purpose, at least for now. When the books have all been written, maybe I will move on to something else, but for now, this is it.

June 20, 2019

I am extremely depressed right now, but I feel myself starting to come out of it. Probably because I have taken my medication. I need to take a shower, and it seems like the hardest task in the world right now. All I really want to do is cry and lay in bed. It's really hard to explain to anyone who hasn't experienced depression. I decided that

I am going to just focus on taking a shower and worry about the rest of my night later. If I can take a shower in the condition I'm in right now, that would really be an accomplishment.

It's not always monumental tasks that I need to accomplish. Sometimes it's the small tasks that seem near impossible. I hate the baby steps approach to depression and anxiety, but that's all I can do when things are bad. Maybe taking a shower will give me the confidence to do something more productive and happy later tonight.

If you asked me why I am depressed right now, I probably couldn't answer that. Depression just exists at times. It's just there, and I don't know how to get out of it right now. I can journal and think of things I'm grateful for. I can just ride it out until my medicine levels me out. I can try every trick in the book, but depression can be immune to all the ways to make me feel better. There's times when nothing helps.

June 21, 2019

Every day I survive is like a giant middle finger to my illness. I'm not bitter or angry at life, but it often helps me to have a chip on my shoulder. If you have a mental illness, be prepared to fight. In order to keep up the fight, I have to get "fired up", because life can get boring and repetitive. Life is just flat out hard too. I don't think this is hard to understand. People mentally prepare themselves all the time to accomplish goals on a daily basis. To use a sports analogy, some of the best victories have come from the underdog because that team had a chip on their shoulder and they felt like the world doubted their success. In my reality, there is no one doubting me, or maybe there is, but in order for me to have the energy to fight, I have to live with a chip on my shoulder and have that fire burning.

Ironically, I take my sense of humor very seriously. What I mean is that if I can laugh through tough times, I feel like I am winning at life. It helps me when I can make others laugh too, even if just for a few moments. My sense of humor is one of the last dignities I have left, and it has never been taken from me when a lot of other things have. I was joking just days out of my first hospitalization. So when people think I am being funny, I am actually fighting very hard to keep a light, kind heart in the midst of hardship and sadness. I get as much from making people laugh as the people I am making laugh do.

June 23, 2019

Today is Sunday. I made a nice recovery from depression on Friday, and I went out to lunch with my mom. We went to the casino in downtown Cincinnati too, which was a victory over my anxiety as well as eating lunch out. I think I had a let down yesterday (Saturday) though. I was just angry and tired all day. Last night, I slept about 6 hours, which is way more than I usually sleep at night. I turned off the lights and social media. All I did was lay in bed and watch golf on TV. It was very relaxing. I didn't want to be around anyone with the attitude that I had, so I guess I isolated myself. I always advocate that everyone should rest when they need to and take care of their mental health, but I forget to do it myself.

June 27, 2019

Yesterday, I mailed a package at the Post Office, picked up a prescription, and got some smoking supplies, all during Rush Hour. Things like this are extremely hard for me because of my anxiety, but I did it with barely any problems. I may not be able to do it tomorrow, but I did it that day. If you talk about material things as blessings, you don't know what a blessing is. THAT was a blessing.

Lately, I have been managing my mood and anxiety better. I try to keep in mind that my extremes never last, and I always come back to a more level mood eventually. I try not to get too excited when things are going well or too depressed when I don't feel well. This is much easier said than done. Depression and mania are very powerful forces and emotions. There's only so much that therapy and medication can do in the name of damage control.

June 29, 2019

I just had a scary experience. It's happened to me before. It's about midnight on a Friday night. I was a little stressed out today, but I'm feeling a little better. Probably my night meds. Anyway, I had a bowel movement, and I started to panic and just feel weird. I was playing games on my computer, and I went out on my porch to have a cigarette. I got really light headed, and I felt like I might pass out. It only lasted a few seconds, but it was scary. One thing I noticed was in those few seconds, a million nonsensical thoughts raced through my mind. None of it made any sense. I had tingling in my arms, head, and chest. After it was over, I felt some relief. Whether it's a panic attack or some other scary experience, I always want to tell everyone that I love them and how much they mean to me. I don't know whether that's a symptom or my personality. A lot of mental illness is like that. What's mental illness and what's my identity. People always say, "You are not your illness", but how true is that?

July 2, 2019

I have a foggy memory of a male nurse, who I swore was the reincarnation of Jerry Garcia. I don't think I believed him when he told me he wasn't in fact Jerry Garcia. When I was psychotic, I used to think I knew everyone and everyone looked familiar. I can't remember if it freaked me out or was comforting. In my defense, I know a lot of people and I come from a small town in Ohio, so seeing familiar people every day isn't unusual. It was unusual because it was everyone, everywhere. I remember my mind operating very quickly. It was almost like my thoughts were flash cards that kept changing at a frantic pace. The thoughts didn't usually make sense, and they changed so rapidly, that I barely had time to process the thoughts anyway.

July 3, 2019

When I was younger, I doubted whether I was actually a strong person. The kind of person who would get back up if I took a punch. I was always hard working and smart, but in really hard times, how would I respond? After dealing with mental illness "officially" for almost 13 years, there is no question that I am a strong person. I answered the bell many times. No matter which version of me you have gotten, I hope I have always been the same person in general. There's just some things about my personality that mental illness never took from me. I'm not saying my life is harder than anyone else's or anything like that, but it's a pretty amazing story. I'm giving it my best shot, and that's all I can do.

July 4, 2019

It's the Fourth of July. I have another foggy memory that is somewhat relevant to Independence Day. I don't remember what year this was, but I remember sitting on my porch, and I felt compelled to take the American flag off the house and march with it. I ripped the flag out from the house, bolts and all, and started marching towards the nearest police station. I don't know exactly what I was thinking, but I think I thought I was trying to show appreciation to the police force by bringing them the flag. My best guess is that I was manic and psychotic at the same time, because I had the energy of mania and the disconnect from reality of psychosis. I remember having so much energy that I walked/marched from my house to the police station in formal shoes, no socks, about 3 miles away. I took a short cut through a park, and a police officer stopped me. I knew the cop from my childhood, and he asked me a few questions. I wasn't doing anything illegal, so I guess that's why he let me go and didn't think anything of it. I know this incident must have been around my worst time, which was 2006, but I rarely have had a manic and psychotic episode at the same time. You can probably imagine how dangerous it would be to be in this state of mind. It was like I had the strength and energy of ten men, and at the same time, it was like someone or something else was at the controls of my rational mind. I can't explain it any better than that. There's a saying about bipolar disorder that goes, "Medication took my superpowers away". That's how I felt that day. Super human.

July 4, 2019

My mom has always cooked dinner every night for the family. My dad went to work, and when he came home, my mom would have dinner ready. This is a tradition that is still alive today, even though it is only my parents and me that live together now. I come from a family of seven; three brothers and a sister.

When I was most sick around this time in 2006, I used to get a sense of calm by watching my mom prepare and cook dinner. I don't know if it was because I was zoned out on medication, or if the monotonous motions were calming to my mind that had endured so much trauma for so long. I still enjoy watching my mom cook dinner, except now, I can pitch in and help, although she usually likes to do it alone. I think cooking dinner satisfies her maternal and nurturing side. She has always been a great mother to me, even when I misbehaved and even when I wasn't so loving or loveable. We have a great relationship now, and I love to make her laugh and make her happy. Her happiness is a priority in my life, and maybe that satisfies the nurturing and caring side of myself.

July 5, 2019

The local and national news are upsetting to me, so I avoid watching at all costs. I happened to see a story today though that struck a chord with me. A man approached police officers in a park with a butcher knife, and he was shot. He is fighting for his life in the hospital. He had no criminal record, but he had a history of mental illness. The story just makes me sad for a few reasons. I know what it's like to be paranoid and feel threatened and have no idea what I was doing. I've never really been violent, but I have done some really strange things and had my run-ins with the police. I had a compassionate judge on two occasions, and instead of jail, I was put into a mental health facility. I'm so lucky that I got help, even though it was pretty much against my will. I just keep thinking that it could have been me so long ago. I'm not defending either side. I don't know what a police officer is supposed to do besides defend himself when a guy is coming at him with a butcher knife. Maybe the violent guy wouldn't get help. But also maybe the mental health system failed him. Just a sad story to me, and it hits close to my heart.

July 8, 2019

I had a very weird experience last night. That's the only way I can describe it. About 5pm, I experienced full body soreness. I can't say for sure whether it was related to my mental illness symptoms. It's very hot outside this time of year, and I'm not in the best shape. Maybe it was something I ate. It was extremely uncomfortable, and all I could do was lay in bed and wait for the pain to stop. I don't take over-the-counter medications of any kind, but I probably should have. It was a long night. When I woke up this morning, I had some coffee as usual, and I couldn't stop sweating. It's about 4am right now, and it's only 70 degrees Fahrenheit outside. It seems odd that I would be sweating so much. Maybe I just needed to rest. I have been going pretty hard lately with this book and other projects. I was thinking the body soreness was some kind of way for my body to express nervous or manic energy. That's why I brought up this incident in the first place.

As I have said before, be prepared to feel weird sometimes with mental illness. Between the side effects of the medication and the symptoms of the actual illness, it's a rough battle most of the time.

July 9, 2019

"Stick to Psalms and Proverbs" said the Christian man in charge of our Bible study group in the hospital. I did for the most part, except I became obsessed with the Book of Revelations and the end of the world in general. This hospital stay was voluntary, and much different than my first hospitalization in 2006. There were board games, arts and crafts, support groups, and even a few exercise machines with a TV. I remember a refrigerator full of cheese wedges and apple juice, which was probably my favorite part. I would get up around 3am and march down the halls with my Bible. I would drink decaf coffee and talk to the nurses at their station. We weren't allowed to have caffeine, which seems like a reasonable idea for mental patients.

I remember laying in my hospital bed and thinking I was on an airplane on the way to see the Pope or maybe the President. I thought I was "the Chosen One", and I still don't know what that means. I thought I was very important, that's for sure. I remember asking for print outs of maps because I thought I could predict earthquakes. I thought a big earthquake was going to hit somewhere and end the Earth. A few days later, an earthquake hit California, but I had predicted one in China, so I thought my prognostication was just a little off. I got these ideas through messages that I thought were from God through the TV, radio, and common items like energy drink can labels and lottery tickets. I thought the thermostat in the hospital controlled everyone's minds. After three days, I checked myself out, and I haven't been back since. This happened around 2008.

July 10, 2019

I really want to tell everyone why I get so emotional this time of year, but that's a surprise at the end of this book. If bipolar disorder can ever been seen as a blessing, it is that I feel things so deeply. It's amazing when I feel happiness, joy, excitement, and compassion so deeply, but the curse of it is also that I feel depression, anxiety, and sadness very deeply as well. There was a time when I was so sedated that I couldn't feel anything. I don't know if there is a worse feeling than feeling numb to everything, especially for people with bipolar disorder, because I just want to be up and manic all the time. Mania feels so good, but it can be so dangerous. Impulsive spending, drugs and alcohol, hyper-sexuality, delusions, and hallucinations are some of mania's calling cards. I also have a brand of bipolar disorder that has psychotic features, which are thoughts and subsequent actions that are a total break from reality and logic. I have gone through psychosis several times, and the easiest way to describe it is that it's like I was watching myself in a movie and someone or something else was at the controls of my mind.

July 14, 2019

I'm trying to read a book right now about a woman with bipolar disorder who wasn't diagnosed until she was 51 years old. I say trying because it's extremely hard for me to focus to read for long periods of time. I have been chipping away at this book just a few pages at a time. It's very interesting because she had a lot of the same symptoms I had---hallucinations, obsessively making lists, extreme irritation, and so much more. It's also interesting because the average age of onset is 24 years old. This is the oldest age of diagnosis I have ever read about, in my limited research about case studies.

Eventually, her symptoms became so severe that she needed to be hospitalized, just like myself. The subject of the book seemed to almost enjoy her stay at the hospital because it was such a slower pace than her normal professional and family life. She talks about it mostly in a fond way. My experiences in the hospital were mostly traumatizing. Maybe I just compare the hospital setting with the freedoms I have in the outside world. I really didn't understand much that was going on while I was in the hospital, which is why I needed to be there in the first place.

July 17, 2019

I think the technical term is disassociation. I just get this weird feelings sometimes where my head feels congested and my mind starts racing. My mind goes from one idea to another very rapidly. Sometimes, the ideas are jumbled and don't even make any sense. It always passes within a few minutes, but I often have to sit down or steady myself against a wall until the feeling passes. It could also be anxiety/panic, so I try to use a technique called grounding to focus my mind. Grounding is focusing on things around you that you can use your senses on. Generally, it usually means staring at stationary objects so my mind can snap back to reality, per se. It's a frightening sensation. My mind can range from nonsensical, jumbled racing thoughts to flashbacks of the hospital and ambulance sirens.

I live on a busy street for the suburbs, and there are sirens often. These sirens used to make me panic and feel squeamish every time an emergency vehicle would drive by. I'm pretty sure the panic was part of having flashbacks, which is why PTSD is part of my complete diagnosis. All of my PTSD symptoms have to do with emergency-type situations and the hospital.

July 18, 2019

I feel so guilty about everything. I feel guilty for everything I put my family and loved ones through with my illness. I feel guilty when I go out and leave the house because what if something happens? What if I end up in the hospital again? What if I wreck my car? What if my loved ones need me while I am out having fun? It would all be my fault, and a part of me feels like my illness is my fault. I read scholarly articles all the time and inspirational blurbs about how mental illness is really no one's fault, but I just can't help to feel responsible.

I went out two nights this week, and it takes me forever to leave the house because getting ready is exhausting. Not only do I have to do all the physical things like get dressed, but I have to overcome the guilt and anxiety that I am feeling. That's why I usually stay home. It's just so exhausting to go out, and taxing on my mind and body.

This is probably my imagination, but I feel like I have to meet high expectations at every moment. I feel like I can never slip up or have a bad day or be in a bad mood. It's an incredible amount of pressure for anyone, much less someone with an illness of extremes and destruction. If I ever get irritated outwardly at someone without good reason, I always apologize. I'm not too big for that. It's a little embarrassing when I can't seem to get a grip on a good mood, or I get upset over something insignificant.

I also feel like my mood has been rapidly cycling, which is usually not a characteristic of my illness, but it is a lot of the time with bipolar disorder. Rapid cycling usually means that a full-blown manic or depressive episode is coming, although some bipolar people just have rapid cycling as a regular symptom. It's exhausting and frustrating to go from low to high so many times in a day.

July 22, 2019

I can't remember when this happened in the sequence of events, but I spent a night in jail in downtown Cincinnati. I got arrested for criminal damaging and trespassing because I got into an unlocked car and tried to start it up. I was psychotic, and I thought this car was a gift from the CIA. I remember it was a Lexus luxury car, but I don't remember damaging anything. I was put in a holding cell with about 15 other men. The size of the cell was about as big as a large broom closet. I remember demanding a phone call, and I threatened to throw my food tray at the guards if I was not granted that right. This is probably when they moved me into my own cell. I got a hold of my mom on the phone and she came down to bail me out. She had to wait several hours until they released me, for some odd reason. I had a trial or court hearing, and I was found not guilty by reason of insanity.

I remember the jail cell that I had to myself. I remember looking out the window at the streets of downtown Cincinnati and wishing I was a free man. The meal the cops brought me was hot dogs, sauerkraut, and white bread. Nothing to drink. I remember I had to ask for water. I don't remember much else about this experience. I know I never want to go back. That's for sure.

Thirteen years ago today, my life was turned upside down...

July 31, 2006 seemed like it would be a regular day. I was working long hours, and using alcohol and marijuana heavily for years. I was barely sleeping. I started having auditory and visual hallucinations as well as delusions, like I was working for the CIA and my house had microphones in it. I thought I could see hidden messages in every day things like lottery tickets and the US mail. I went to my parents' house because I was following one of these hidden messages to do so. My brother was there, and he convinced me to lay down, and I heard something like a freight train between my ears. I thought God was talking to me or maybe angels. It was almost as if I could feel my brain cracking open. Doctors call this a "first break" of bipolar disorder, which seems appropriate now.

The doctors said I suffered a brain trauma similar to a car accident victim. After receiving a large dose of medicine in a large syringe and sleeping for several hours, I was escorted to a locked down psychiatric unit at University Hospital in Cincinnati for 11 days until I was no longer a harm to myself or others.

I went through psychosis, which is a total break from reality. I had a few other hospitalizations, but none were as severe as in 2006, and I haven't been hospitalized since around 2010. I have PTSD as a result of my hospitalizations because I saw some terrible things and the whole experience is burned into my memory.

I remember being surrounded by nurses and police officers, and one of the nurses was holding a large syringe full of medicine. I was psychotic and panicking. Eventually, I allowed the nurse to plunge the needle deep into my arm. Within minutes, I felt the medicine working. I slept in a little room away from the main area for a really long time. Honestly, it was the best sleep I had in years.

Another terrible memory of this hospitalization was seeing a naked man on a stretcher who was being forced to take medicine. I don't know what the situation was, but the man was shrieking in terror. That image is burned into my mind, as well as an image of a large syringe. When I have flashbacks related to PTSD, these images are usually the ones that come to mind. I also have flashbacks about riding in ambulances many times, and also flashbulb memories of when I was psychotic. It's all a little blurry as you can probably imagine.

Afterword

I hope this collection of thoughts and journal entries has helped you in some way, whether it be a better understanding of mental illness, or not feeling alone with your own illness. I want to thank my entire support system including, doctors, nurses, family and friends, and you, the reader. I would not have made it this far without tons of loving support. Peace and love to you all.

Made in the USA
Columbia, SC
22 October 2020